Alzh

PROTECTIN

What Ou ... ... Didn't Know

Dr. Melody Jemison

Copyright © 2012

Dr. Melody Jemison

All rights reserved.

www.nomorealzheimers.com

www.alzheimerspreventionlifestyle.com

dr.melodyjemison@gmail.com

Table of Contents

Chapter 1 Introduction

It was the first time my father did not recognize me.

"Have you met Melody?" he asked, looking directly at me.

Stunned, I replied, "Yes. I've met her once or twice."

"Well," he continued. "You two are so much alike that I don't think you would get along at all!"

Wow! Sad as the moment was, I just had to throw back my head and laugh at the irony of it. God bless him! What can you say to that?

Then the realization sank in. My grandmother died with Alzheimer's. Now my dad has it and three of his four siblings have it. Am I next? What about my brother and my nine cousins on that side of the family? Will it continue to the next generation? What about my daughter and grandson? Alzheimer's disease felt like a freight train bearing down on me. What could I do?

I began a search to learn what was known about Alzheimer's prevention. I immersed myself in research studies, summaries, abstracts, full length papers and interpretations of these studies.

I was shocked at what I found.

My conclusion after all this searching is that **YES, Alzheimer's disease is preventable**. It is primarily a lifestyle disease, much like type 2 diabetes. There are genetic factors that change your inherent risk. **However, if you do the right things at the right times in your life, you can still reduce your chances of developing Alzheimer's to near zero!**

In writing this book, I put together a compilation of summary articles that explain the research in layman's terms. Whenever possible, I used research interpretations that summarized the results in a percentage of risk reduced or increased. For example, one study showed **that people who drank fruit and vegetable juices more than three times a week were 76% less likely to develop Alzheimer's disease than those who drank juices less than once a week.**[1]

Wow! That's a huge number and it is only one of **27 specific recommendations backed by research**. My premise is simple. The more of these recommendations you incorporate into your lifestyle, the healthier your body and brain will be, thus dramatically reducing your risk of developing Alzheimer's.

So why haven't we heard about this? That's a good question. My feeling is that "prevention" does not make much money. That may be cynical, but I believe it to be the true motive. There are a few lone voices out there seeking to educate the public about Alzheimer's prevention. I now join with them and hope that as you read and learn, you will be excited to share it with others, too.

Alzheimer's is a cruel disease. Not only does it rob us of our memories, but of our very life – the core of who we are. One in 8 older Americans has Alzheimer's and it is the 6th leading cause of death in the United States, according to the Alzheimer's Association's web site at www.alz.org.[2]

At the time of this writing, there is no known cure for Alzheimer's. Once symptoms begin, the usual disease process leads to memory loss, mental impairment and ultimately, death. Children are robbed of their grandparents, spouses of their partners, and families watch a cherished loved one slowly slip away much sooner than necessary.

3

To make matters worse, some families can't seem to get away from it. My grandmother had Alzheimer's. She was one of 13 children. Many of her siblings had Alzheimer's and now, 4 of her 5 children have it.

There are several genes associated with Alzheimer's disease. The most common is called ApoE4. If you have one copy of this gene (from one parent), you are 3 times more likely to develop dementia than someone who does not have the gene. If you inherited 2 copies of the gene (one from each parent), you are 10 times more likely to develop the disease.[3] That's scary when you know it runs in your family. I was really excited to find that these recommendations helped even those with a family history of the disease.

This, my friends, is very good news; worthy of sharing with everyone you care about. You see, **anyone can develop Alzheimer's, with or without the susceptibility genes.** No one, that lives long enough, is completely immune, unless they know what to do to prevent it! And, if you wait until you are older and starting to show symptoms — it may be too late to make a significant difference at that point.

Prevention best begins early. The sooner, the better. Pathological changes in the brain can start developing 20-30 years before the symptoms of mental decline and memory loss begin. I have a full set of recommendations based on research that will help you protect and even improve your brain function.

I believe in a holistic approach to health and healing. Therefore, my program includes recommendations for your body, mind and spirit. These three aspects of our selves are so intertwined and overlapping that they cannot be separated. To ignore one aspect can be detrimental to the others.

My style of writing for this book is simple and easy to understand. I wrote it in simple language as if we were having a kitchen table discussion. I've included a number of well written articles or portions of articles that explain the research in easy to understand terms. I've added bold emphasis for important conclusions.

Because I believe in a holistic and organic approach, some of my recommendations go against current Western medical advice. However, the research I share supports the positions I advocate. All references are given with internet links. You can research it for yourself, if you are so inclined.

At this point in the introduction, I would normally give the standard medical disclaimer. However, my disclaimer has a disclaimer. *Any and all information given in this book is not intended as medical advice, but given only for information.* That much is true.

However, the second part to the medical disclaimer is, *if you have questions about the information contained in this book and its relevance to you, consult your medical doctor.* Yes, you should discuss anything with your doctor that concerns your health and/or your medications. However, your medical doctor may or may not have a detailed knowledge of nutrition and supplements.

Medical doctors in the United States have a "medicine" and "disease/sickness" focus, in other words, a *"pill for every ill"* mentality; not one of prevention, health and nutrition. Therefore, I urge you to educate yourself about these things and take responsibility for your own health. Truly, no one else can do that for you, not even your medical doctor.

Be educated and informed about health issues that may affect you. Partner with your doctor concerning your health goals. I know some medical doctors cringe when they hear someone say this. They accurately point out there is much misinformation "out there" on the internet. That is true, but there also is a wealth of accurate information on-line.

In fact, you can peruse *www.PubMed.com.* for research information on almost every subject imaginable. PubMed.com was developed by the U.S. National Library of Medicine and contains over 2.2 million items. You can search the site for any word or phrase such as, *Alzheimer's disease* or *memory loss* or *Alzheimer's prevention.* However, without a medical background, you may get frustrated trying to read the scientific and medical lingo.

Fortunately, there are many reputable sources like the *Mayo Clinic, Livestrong.com, and the National Institutes of Health,* who have medical writers to read and "translate" the reports into plain English that's easy to understand. Their articles are referenced. You can go back and look at the original research paper for yourself.

I noticed something very interesting when I read different articles giving interpretations about the same study. Some writers would present it in a positive, promising light and others would downplay the information, warning readers not to "get their hopes up".

For example, in one of the rat studies, a supplement was tested that caused great mental and physical improvement on maze tests. One writer was excited about what this could mean for humans and presented the findings in a hopeful positive light. Another writer basically said, "Don't get too excited. These are rats, not humans. We still don't have any conclusive results from human, double blind, long term studies that prove anything for us."

Well, that may be. However, rats are used in labs for good reasons. One being, that results from rat studies help researchers design the next step needed in a human study.

My opinion is that if we wait around for all of the double blind, long term, human use studies to be done and replicated before we adapt and recommend those changes – it could be too late. And if the recommendation will not harm you anyway, then why on earth wait? Another generation or two could die with Alzheimer's while the studies are waiting to happen.

It made me sad to see doctor after doctor say that we do not have "conclusive research" of anything definitive that will prevent Alzheimer's. If you only look at one study at a time, that may be true and it could depend on your definition of "conclusive research".

However, I believe that when you see all of the studies I have detailed in this book, you will agree **there is an overwhelming preponderance of evidence showing that we can greatly lower our risk of developing Alzheimer's to the point of prevention.**

Therefore, instead of facing the prospects of this devastating disease of Alzheimer's with fear, I now feel empowered to change the course of my future. I hope you will join me.

My heart still sorrows for those, like my dad, who are already affected to the point they will not likely recover. We do still need a cure. I support on-going Alzheimer's research and will continue to participate in fundraising and awareness projects. Please visit my web site at www.nomorealzheimers.com for more information and know that a percentage of the profits of this book will go toward continued research for a cure.

* Note – all **BOLD** in this book has been added by author for emphasis.

Chapter 2

What is Alzheimer's disease?

Alzheimer's disease is an irreversible, progressive brain disease that slowly destroys memory and thinking skills. Even the ability to carry out the simplest tasks of daily living is eventually destroyed. Symptoms of the disease usually appear after age 60. The average age is 65. Alzheimer's disease is the most common cause of dementia among older people, according to the National Institute of Aging.[1]

Although currently without a clear-cut diagnostic model, Alzheimer's is associated with **degeneration of brain cells called neurons.** Brain cells communicate with each other via chemical neurotransmitters. One of the most active is acetylcholine. However, as neurons degenerate, the amount of **acetylcholine in the brain is decreased.** Other pathological changes seen in an Alzheimer's brain includes abnormal clumps called **beta-amyloid plagues**, and tangled fibers called neurofibrillary tangles, or **tau tangles**.

This process begins in the region of the brain associated with memory and eventually spreads to other areas effecting language, balance, mood, behavior and bodily functions. As brain cells degenerate and die off, **the brain actually begins to shrink.**

The cause of Alzheimer's disease is still hotly debated. Many theories exist. Some believe the plagues, tangles and decreased neurotransmitters are the cause of the deterioration. Other neuroscientists believe that the plagues and tangles are a result (or side effect) of the unknown cause. Part of the problem is that as we age everyone has plagues and tangles to some degree. Generally, people with Alzheimer's have more of these brain changes than those without the disease.

To confuse the matter even more is the fact that **some people with larger amounts of plagues and tangles still function fairly well mentally.** Clearly, more research is needed to understand this complex disease process. However, we can still benefit from research that has been done.

My focus in reviewing this research has been prevention. What can I do to prevent from following my family's genetic footsteps? I formulated my conclusions in the **No More**

Alzheimer's Prevention Plan. In it are many recommendations to greatly decrease our risk of Alzheimer's, allowing us to protect our brains.

Picture a frail elderly person. They may be tiny; much smaller than they were in the prime of their lives. Year by year, their height decreases. Muscles atrophy and shrink. Getting around requires a walker. Weakened, the smallest task takes effort. Life is difficult. Eyesight has dimmed. Hearing is diminished. Memory is failing to the point of not recognizing family. Millions of families have lived this sad scenario.

Now, picture a strong, healthy senior citizen. Their frame may have shrunk slightly from its previous size. However, they still have a sparkle in their eyes and spunk in their personality. They can walk for blocks and play a mean game of checkers. They make it a point to be active and eat nutritious food. Full of energy with a passion for life, they easily laugh and keep a positive frame of mind. Friends, family and faith are important. They may be aging, yet they still look forward to the future.

What causes this great divergence in quality of life? Some are so vibrant, healthy and strong; others are feeble, weak and depressed. Why? Are some just lucky? We could assume they have good genetics. But, most healthy senior citizens have made good decisions along the way. They've made their health a priority, including what they eat, how they exercise, staying socially active and finding a way to still enjoy life.

The first of the baby boomer generation has now reached retirement. The percentage of the population over age 65 is increasing and will continue for many years. However, with this increase comes additional health care expense. Health care costs in general are soaring. Caring for patients with Alzheimer's is very expensive. Many experts use the word "tsunami" to describe the expected increase in cases of Alzheimer's disease in the near future. **Some research suggests the number of Alzheimer's patients could triple — some say quadruple — by 2050.**[2]

There is good news. I believe that by the time you finish reading this book, you will be convinced that Alzheimer's disease is preventable. **If we can delay the onset of Alzheimer's symptoms by <u>one year</u>, then**

13

210,000 people will be saved from this terrible disease. If that happens, it has been estimated that the accumulated savings would be nearly $10 billion in health care costs over a 10 year time period in the United States.[3] That is a significant difference in terms of lives affected, as well as dollars saved.

Research shows that it is never too late to make positive improvements. For example, in a series of independently conducted studies on the effects of exercise in healthy older adults, it was confirmed that spending time at the gym not only maintains good health but helps prevent the onset of chronic diseases, including heart disease, osteoarthritis and dementia.

In one of the studies sited, scientists in Germany found that **increased physical activity was associated with a lower incidence of dementia.** In this study, 3,485 elderly people were asked about their physical activity. None of the participants had dementia at the start of the analysis, but after two years of follow-up, researchers found **that those who exercised at least three times a week were half as likely to have developed** dementia,[4] as those who reported no physical activity.

In the following chapters, I detail an easy to follow plan that you can customize to your personal goals. You will be amazed at the information presented. Anyone can follow this plan.

There is hope for a future without Alzheimer's disease. The answer and the ability to choose our future is in our hands. We now have the knowledge that our parents and grandparents did not have. My grandmother lived her final years in an "Alzheimer's cottage" with 24 hour, around the clock supervision. I look forward to the time when that cottage and all such nursing facilities are vacant. Join me to create a future without Alzheimer's!

Chapter 3   Nutrition

"The doctor of the future will give no medicine, but will interest his patients in the care of the human frame, in a proper diet, and in the cause and prevention of disease."
Thomas Edison

Quality nutrition is the cornerstone of the *No More Alzheimer's Prevention Plan*. A healthy diet consisting of fresh fruits, vegetables, adequate protein and quality fats will benefit both brain and body. However, the brain has very specific nutritional requirements that are often lacking in the average American diet. When the brain is given the nutrients it needs, it can function very well, even into the later years of life.

Hectic lifestyles make fast foods and processed foods the primary choice of many households.   We are conditioned to eat "comfort" food during stressful times. The web site *Sixwise.com* reports the following:

Every day, 7 percent of the U.S. population visits a McDonald's, and 20-25 percent eats fast food of some kind, says Steven Gortmaker, professor of Society, Human development, and Health at the Harvard School of Public Health. As for children, 30 percent between the ages of 4 and 19 eat fast food on any given day.

But that's just the tip of the iceberg. Americans get processed food not only from fast-food restaurants but also from their neighborhood grocery stores. **As it stands, about 90 percent of the money that Americans spend on food is used to buy — that's right — processed foods.**[1]

As a result, our nation is getting fatter, sicker, weaker and suffering more mental decline as we age. To reverse this trend, we must change the way we look at food and understand the long term consequences of our choices.

Everyone knows being overweight increases your risk for cardiovascular disease, heart attacks and strokes, diabetes and even some forms of cancer. **But did you know that being overweight also puts you at greater risk for Alzheimer's and other dementias?**[2]

Therefore, to protect your brain long term, you must reach and maintain your healthiest weight. It gives me a little extra motivation to realize that eating cookies or chips not only hurt my health, but also increase my risk of developing Alzheimer's.

Antioxidants

What makes for a diet that not only helps keep your brain from deteriorating, but also helps build new brain cells and strengthen existing ones? Let's start with **antioxidants**. According to the Franklin Institute:

> Oxygen makes life possible, but it can also take life away. Each of your hundred-billion brain cells uses oxygen to function. Your brain's need for oxygen is more than ten times greater than the rest of your body. This same oxygen, however, can also erode the very structure of those brain cells. Highly-reactive forms of oxygen called free radicals create chemical reactions that damage brain cells. If free radicals get out of control, cells will be damaged faster than they can be repaired. Like a biological form of rust, a lifetime of oxidative insult can lead to diminished brain function. To counteract these radical oxidants, the brain needs an ample supply of antioxidants.[3]

The average American diet contains less than half the recommended daily amount of antioxidants. Several studies have indicated that a diet high in antioxidants may lower the risk of Alzheimer's.[4] Antioxidants are found primarily in fruits, vegetables, spices, coffee and chocolate. What specific foods are high in antioxidants?

The top food group for antioxidants is **berries**! All types of berries, but especially those dark in color. Blueberries, blackberries, cranberries, strawberries, raspberries and elderberries are excellent. Topping the list is acai berries, followed by blueberries and blackberries.

Several common spices are high in antioxidants including cloves, oregano, rosemary, thyme and cinnamon.

Many vegetables score high in antioxidants, especially broccoli, red cabbage, red leaf lettuce, asparagus, and purple cauliflower. Some nuts are also high in antioxidants, including pecans and almonds.

Every morning, I have the same breakfast, just because I like it so much and I know how good it is for my brain and body. I start with about 1/2 cup of cottage cheese. Next, I add 1/2 cup of blueberries, 1/2 cup of blackberries and 1/2 cup of strawberries. I top it with some honey roasted sliced almonds. It is so delicious, I feel like I'm eating candy. I am — nature's candy! I usually have 2 cups of coffee topped with cinnamon, nutmeg and allspice.

Juices

We have been told for years to avoid juices due to naturally occurring high sugar content and lack of fiber. However, juice may be very helpful in protecting the brain from deterioration. *Alzheimer's Weekly* reports the following:

In a study lead by Dr. Richard Hartman, PhD, an assistant professor of psychology at Loma Linda University's School of Science and Technology, found **that a daily glass of pomegranate juice could halve the build-up of harmful proteins linked to Alzheimer's disease.** In fact, his study has shown that **pomegranates work just as well as pharmaceutical medicines.**

Dr. Hartman also collaborated with Washington University researchers on this project. The study began with transgenic mice predisposed to develop Alzheimer's-like pathology and symptoms. At a young age, the mice were split into two groups—half received water with added pomegranate-juice concentrate, and the control group received drinking water with the same amount of sugar as the juice. Dr. Hartman's research found that the mice that drank the pomegranate juice had 50 percent less beta-amyloid plaques in the hippocampus of their brains. The mice drank an average of 5 milliliters of fluid a day, which is roughly equivalent to a human drinking one to two glasses of pomegranate juice a day.[5]

Citing another study on *WebMD.com*, author Jennifer Warner wrote the following:

A new study shows drinking **apple juice may improve memory by preventing the decline of an essential neurotransmitter known as acetylcholine**. Neurotransmitters are chemicals released by nerve cells to transmit messages to other nerve cells. They are critical for good memory and brain health. Previous studies have shown that increasing the amount of acetylcholine in the brain can slow the mental decline found in people with Alzheimer's disease.

In the study, researchers compared normal adult mice, normal "aged" mice, and special mice that were a genetic model for human Alzheimer's. The mice were given either a normal diet, or a diet lacking in essential nutrients, for one month. Some of the mice on the nutrient-poor diet were also given apple juice concentrate mixed in their water.

The results showed that normal adult mice and the genetically-engineered mice on normal diets had the same acetylcholine levels. In fact, the normal adults had the same acetylcholine levels regardless of diet. However, the genetically engineered mice on the nutrient-poor diet had lower acetylcholine levels. **But this drop was prevented in those given apple juice.** In the aged mice on a normal diet, acetylcholine levels were lower than in the normal adult mice; and their levels were even lower if placed on the nutrient-poor diet. But, again, this decline was prevented by the addition of apple juice to drink.

The mice were also put through maze memory tests. "It was surprising how the animals on the apple-enhanced diets actually did a superior job on the maze tests than those not on the supplemented diet," says Shea. **The amount of apple juice the mice drank was comparable to drinking about two 8-ounce glasses of apple juice or eating two to three apples a day for humans.**[6]

One more juice study reported on *WebMD.com*:

Drinking fruit or vegetable juice every other day may keep Alzheimer's disease away. **A new study shows people who drank fruit and vegetable juices more than three times a week were 76% less likely to develop Alzheimer's disease than those who drank juices less than once a week.** Researchers say the results suggest that a class of antioxidants found in fruit and vegetable juices called polyphenols may have a protective effect on the brain and help fight dementia and Alzheimer's disease.

In the study, published in The American Journal of Medicine, researchers followed nearly 2,000 Japanese-American adults from King County, Wash., for 10 years. The participants were aged 65 or older and were free of signs of Alzheimer's or dementia at the start of the study. Self-reported dietary information was obtained from 1,589 of the adults. The average age of this group was 72 years at the start of the study.

Previous studies show Japanese adults living in Japan have a lower incidence of Alzheimer's disease. But Japanese people living in the U.S. have higher rates of the disease, which suggests that environmental factors such as diet and lifestyle may play an important role in the development of Alzheimer's disease.

In addition, the study showed the protective benefits of juice appeared to be particularly enhanced in people who had a genetic marker linked to an increased risk of Alzheimer's disease known as apolipoprotein E å-4 allele (ApoE-4).[7]

Good Fats and Bad Fats

Fat is necessary for energy supply as well as storage and delivery of fat soluble vitamins like A, D and E. Some fats are more beneficial than others. Trans fats have been hotly debated. While popular with the food industry, they have been proven detrimental to our health, including the brain. What are trans fats and how do we get them in our diet?

Trans fats, also called trans fatty acids, are created by adding hydrogen to vegetable oil in a process called hydrogenation. Trans fats make oil less likely to spoil. Trans fats in manufactured foods help products stay fresh and have longer shelf life. They are often found in commercially baked foods including crackers, cookies, cakes, candies and fried foods.[8]

Reading food labels will reveal the amount of trans fats in a product. The total fat listed in grams is located in the upper middle section. Just under the total fat listing are the two categories of saturated fats and trans fats. If trans fats are in the product, it will be listed there. You will also find it listed in the ingredients section as **partially hydrogenated oil**. Due to bad press, many companies have now eliminated trans fats from their food products completely. According to a report on *CBN News*, we learn the following:

Dr. Gene Bowman, of Portland's Oregon Health and Science University, led a study of 104 seniors with an average age of 87. After analyzing blood samples, MRI brain scans and memory test results, he discovered that **the seniors with the highest levels of trans fats in their blood had smaller brains.**

A person's brain size can change with aging. Brain shrinkage is one of the hallmarks of Alzheimer's disease. A larger brain is considered to be healthier. **"We know that in Alzheimer's disease that the brain shrinks at an accelerated pace** as the disease and pathology spreads to certain parts of the brain," Dr. Bowman explained. "But if you have a larger brain and more brain tissue, you might have a reserve to handle that pathology better," he added. **In addition to smaller brains, people who ate more trans fats also scored lower on thinking and memory tests.**[9]

Saturated fat (saturated fatty acids), can also be detrimental to our health. High fat beef, milk and cheese, all contain saturated fat, as well as vegetable oils that are liquid at room temperature. Like trans fats, the amount of saturated fats can be found on product food labels.

ABC Science News out of Australia relates the following report connecting saturated fats and Alzheimer's:

Australian researchers believe they have discovered why foods high in saturated fat increase the likelihood of developing Alzheimer's disease. Researchers from Curtin University of Technology in Perth found that **saturated dietary fat damages the lining of blood vessels in the brains of mice, allowing a protein called amyloid to enter the brain.**

The study, to be published in the *British Journal of Nutrition*, is one of the first to demonstrate a scientific link between diet and Alzheimer's disease. "In the past population studies suggested that high fat diets may be a risk factor for Alzheimer's disease, but no one really understood why," says Professor Mamo, co-author of the study and National Director of the Australian Technology Network's Centre for Metabolic Fitness.

The brain has millions of blood vessels. Each vessel has a lining that is very selective about what is allowed to go in and out, and this keeps the brain in good health." Mamo and colleagues found this lining, called the blood-brain-barrier, is damaged by high saturated fat diets. "This allows things to be getting in there that shouldn't be," says Mamo.

A key feature of Alzheimer's disease is amyloid deposits in the brain, which cause inflammation and nerve cell death. Amyloid is produced in the small intestine, and secreted into the blood where it attacks the blood-brain-barrier. "When the blood vessel lining

25

gets disrupted and deregulated you get delivery of amyloid into the brain," says Mamo.[10]

Just as saturated fats are detrimental to our health, **unsaturated fats are beneficial.** Included in this category are **polyunsaturated fatty acids and monounsaturated fats.** Polyunsaturated fats, found mostly in vegetable oils, also include the omega-3 fatty acids, popular for their heart-health benefits. **Omega-3s are found in fatty fish** (salmon, trout, catfish, mackerel) and flaxseed and walnuts.

Monounsaturated fats are typically liquid at room temperature and found in olives, avocados, hazelnuts, almonds, Brazil nuts, cashews, sesame seeds and pumpkin seeds, as well as and olive, canola, and peanut oils.

In a study reported in the *Archives of Neurology,* we find the following:

Researchers at Rush-Presbyterian St. Luke's Medical Center in Chicago studied 815 nursing home residents aged 65 and older for seven years. None had Alzheimer's at the start of the study in 1993; though 131 went on to develop Alzheimer's during the trial. **Men and women who reported eating fish at least once a week had a 60 percent lower risk of getting Alzheimer's compared to those who rarely or almost never ate fish.** "Our findings suggest that consumption of fish—at least weekly—may reduce the risk of Alzheimer's disease," concluded Martha Clare Morris, a lead author of the study.[11]

The bottom line is to understand the difference between "good and bad" fats. Read food labels and know what you are putting in your mouth. Limit your consumption of trans and saturated fats. Add good fats to protect your heart and brain.

Coffee, Tea and Water

In a recent study of the effect of blood caffeine levels, it was found that **older adults who drank the equivalent of 3-4 cups of coffee per day were protected from developing Alzheimer's**. According to the *Journal of Alzheimer's Disease*, researchers from the University of South Florida and the University of Miami say the case control study provides the first direct evidence of caffeine and reduced risk of dementia. The collaborative study involved 124 people, ages 65 to 88, in Tampa and Miami.

These intriguing results suggest that older adults with mild memory impairment who drink moderate levels of coffee — about 3 cups a day — will not convert to Alzheimer's disease, or at least will experience a substantial delay before converting to Alzheimer's," said study lead author Dr. Chuanhai Cao, a neuroscientist at the USF College of Pharmacy and the USF Health Byrd Alzheimer's Institute. "The results from this study, along with our earlier studies in Alzheimer's mice, are very consistent in indicating that moderate daily caffeine/coffee intake throughout adulthood should appreciably protect against Alzheimer's disease later in life.

The study shows this protection probably occurs even in older people with early signs of the disease, called mild cognitive impairment, or MCI. Patients with MCI already experience some short-term memory loss and initial Alzheimer's pathology in their brains. Each year, about 15 percent of MCI patients progress to full-blown Alzheimer's disease. The researchers focused on study participants with MCI, because many were destined to develop Alzheimer's within a few years.[12]

Livestrong.com reports the following results regarding different types of tea, cola and coffee:

In the February 2006 issue of *The American Journal of Clinical Nutrition* researchers analyzed the beverage consumption patterns of 1,003 Japanese subjects with an average age of 74. The beverages included green, black and oolong tea, coffee, cola and 100 percent vegetable juice. **The researchers found that people who drank more than two cups of green tea per day had a 50 percent lower incidence of cognitive impairment.** EGCG, or epigallocatechin gallate, is an antioxidant found in green tea that researchers frequently study for its health benefits.

German researchers reporting in the June 2008 issue of *Nature Structural & Molecular Biology* discovered a way in which EGCG may benefit Alzheimer's patients. Amyloid plaque is a tangle of proteins commonly seen in the brains of Alzheimer's patients. The accumulation of these proteins creates communication problems between brain cells, resulting in damaged memory function. **The researchers used EGCG to effectively untangle the proteins and restore the pristine state of brain tissue.**

Researchers reporting in the September 2008 issue of *Journal of Nutritional Biochemistry* tested the EGCG connection to Alzheimer's in a rat study. One group of rats received drinking water supplemented with EGCG, while the other received no tea extract. After 26 weeks, the researchers tested the rats' learning ability in a maze.

Twenty weeks later, the rats receiving the EGCG were infused with beta-amyloid protein to prompt formation of the amyloid plagues characteristic of Alzheimer's. After running the animals through the maze and laboratory analysis, **the researchers confirmed that EGCG provided significant protection against amyloid plague formation.** [13]

Water is essential for our health and in particular for our brains. Properly hydrated, the brain's water content is about 85% by weight. When we are dehydrated, our thinking, also called cognitive processes, slow down. Chronic dehydration can even lead to brain shrinkage, as often seen in the elderly and those with Alzheimer's.

In a recent study, researchers also found the participants had to exert much more mental effort to perform certain functions when they were dehydrated, than when they were properly hydrated.[14] Make sure you drink at least 64 oz. of pure drinking water (preferably not tap water) per day. I like to add lemon juice to mine.

If you drink well water, make sure it is tested regularly and know what is in it. Another eco-friendly alternative to purchasing bottled water, is using a simple filtration pitcher like those made by Brita or Pur.

Controlling Blood Sugar

Keeping blood sugar levels within healthy limits is important for our bodies and our brains. **Research now shows that type 2 diabetes increases the risk for Alzheimer's disease**. The *Mayo Clinic* web site tells us the following:

Diabetes and Alzheimer's disease are connected in ways that still aren't completely understood. While not all research confirms the connection, many studies indicate that **people with diabetes — especially type 2 diabetes — are at higher risk of eventually developing Alzheimer's disease. Taking steps to**

prevent or control diabetes may help reduce your risk of Alzheimer's disease.

Because diabetes damages blood vessels, it has long been recognized as a risk factor for vascular dementia — a type of cognitive decline caused by damaged blood vessels in the brain. Many people with cognitive decline have brain changes that are hallmarks of both Alzheimer's disease and vascular dementia. Some researchers think that each condition helps fuel the damage caused by the other. [15]

Type 2 Diabetes is primarily a lifestyle disease. It is caused by overconsumption of simple carbohydrates and processed foods, such as sugar, flour, rice, potatoes, pasta, bread, candy and soft drinks. Diabetes can be caused by chronic imbalance of carbohydrates to proteins and good fats.

This eating pattern leads to an overproduction of the hormone insulin, whose function is to reduce blood sugar (glucose). Insulin is a fat storing hormone. As we produce more fat, we have less available insulin receptors. This prompts the body to try to produce more insulin, but may have trouble keeping up with the demand, due to too many carbohydrates in the diet. The result is a condition called insulin resistance, the precursor to type 2 diabetes.

Type 2 Diabetes can be reversed. The first step is to reduce simple carbohydrates (listed above). Eat more complex carbohydrates instead, such as fruits, vegetables and limited whole grains. Add good quality, lower fat protein with each meal and a small amount of good fats. This balance keeps insulin production at a lower healthy level, making it much easier to clear excess glucose from the blood.

The Mediterranean Diet, Zone Diet, South Beach Diet, Body for Life and Paleo Diets are good eating plans, balancing complex carbohydrates with good quality low fat proteins and healthy fats. You can prevent and/or reverse diabetes while losing weight. Be careful with very low carb diets such as Atkins. It's great for insulin control and weight loss, but may not be good for the cardiovascular system.

Each diet has its pros and cons. Most people know from experience what type diet works best for them. Type 2 diabetes is often cured simply exercising and obtaining your ideal weight.

Alzheimer's is being called "Diabetes Type 3" by some researchers. The web site, *Diabetesincontrol.com* gives the following report:

Researchers at Rhode Island Hospital and Brown Medical School have discovered that some insulin and its related proteins are produced in the brain, and that reduced levels of both are linked to Alzheimer's disease.

What we found is that insulin is not just produced in the pancreas, but also in the brain. And we discovered that insulin and its growth factors, which are necessary for the survival of brain cells, contribute to the progression of Alzheimer's," says senior author Suzanne M. de la Monte, a neuropathologist at Rhode Island Hospital and a professor of pathology at Brown Medical School. "This raises the possibility of a Type 3 diabetes."

It has previously been known that insulin resistance, a characteristic of diabetes, is tied to neurodegeneration. While scientists have suspected a link between diabetes and Alzheimer's disease, this is the first study to provide evidence of that connection.[16]

One of the best ways to protect your brain from Alzheimer's is to reduce your simple carbohydrates and get adequate good quality protein and fats. Pairing protein with carbohydrates helps maintain healthy insulin levels.

Whey protein can be a good option for those who prefer to limit meat. Each morning I fill a 32 oz. drinking bottle with 100 grams of good quality whey protein powder. I add water, shake and sip it throughout the day, knowing I have sufficient protein to balance my carbs. The extra protein completely reduces my carb cravings and appetite. Whey protein comes in different flavors. It's a great tool for anyone needing to lose weight and/or control their insulin production.

Ketones and Coconut Oil

Coconut oil has been touted to help prevent Alzheimer's and even reverse symptoms. The web site *Mercola.com* gives the following detailed explanation of how this may work:

> Dr. Mary Newport writes about ketone bodies, an alternative fuel for your brain which your body makes when digesting coconut oil, and how coconut oil may offer profound benefits in the fight against Alzheimer's disease. If her theory is accurate, this could be one of the greatest natural health discoveries in a long time. Backing up her claims is the remarkable recovery of her own husband.

> "Brain starvation" is a hallmark of Alzheimer's disease. One of the primary fuels your brain needs is glucose, which is converted into energy. The mechanism for glucose uptake in your brain has only recently begun to be studied, and what has been learned is that your brain

actually manufactures its own insulin to convert glucose in your blood stream into the food it needs to survive.

Now, when your brain's production of insulin decreases, your brain literally begins to starve, as it's deprived of the glucose-converted energy it needs to function normally. **This is what happens to Alzheimer's patients — portions of their brain start to atrophy, or starve, leading to impaired functioning and eventual loss of memory, speech, movement and personality.**

In effect, your brain can begin to atrophy from starvation if it becomes insulin resistant and loses its ability to convert glucose into energy. It is now also known that diabetics have a 65 percent increased risk of also being diagnosed with Alzheimer's disease, and there appears to be a potent link between the two diseases, even though the exact mechanisms have yet to be determined. It seems quite clear however that both are related to insulin resistance in your body and in your brain.

Fortunately, your brain is able to run on more than one type of energy supply, and this is where coconut oil enters the picture. There's another substance that can feed your brain and prevent brain atrophy. **It may even restore and renew neuron and nerve function in your brain after damage has set in.** The substance in question is called **ketone bodies**, or ketoacids.

Ketones are what your body produces when it converts fat (as opposed to glucose) into energy. A primary source of ketone bodies are the medium chain triglycerides (MCT) found in coconut oil! Coconut oil contains about 66 percent MCTs.

Another way to increase ketone production in your body is by restricting carbohydrates. This is what happens when you go on a high fat, high protein, low carbohydrate diet: Your body begins to run on fats instead of carbohydrates, and the name for this is ketosis. This is also why you don't starve to death when you restrict food for weeks at a time, because your body is able to convert stored fat into ketones that are used as fuel instead of glucose.

Consuming medium chain triglycerides such as coconut oil is a better option, however, because the ketones produced by ketosis are not concentrated in your bloodstream, but are instead mostly excreted in your urine.

Therapeutic levels of MCTs have been studied at 20 grams per day. According to Dr. Newport's calculations, just over two tablespoons of coconut oil (about 35 ml or 7 level teaspoons) would supply you with the equivalent of 20 grams of MCT, which is indicated as either a preventative measure against degenerative neurological diseases, or as a treatment for an already established case.

Remember though that people tolerate coconut oil differently, and you may have to start slowly and build up to these therapeutic levels. My recommendation is to start with one teaspoon, taken with food in the mornings. Gradually add more coconut oil every few days until you are able to tolerate four tablespoons. Coconut oil is best taken with food, to avoid upsetting your stomach."[17]

Personally, I do not like using coconut oil except for cooking. I tried it several ways and just couldn't stomach it, so to speak. I was delighted to find a milk substitute that combines coconut milk (which does contain the medium chain triglycerides) and almond milk. The name is Almond Breeze, made by the Blue Diamond Almond Company. It's an excellent source of calcium and protein. I love the taste and use it in my coffee. Almond Breeze comes in sweetened and unsweetened versions. It's dairy-free and low carbohydrate, as it does not contain milk sugar. Find it in the dairy section of your grocery store.

NutriBullet

I've recently acquired a small kitchen appliance called the *NutriBullet*. My husband and I use it daily. It's similar to a blender and a juicer, but much smaller and easier to use. It's the only product I've found that actually breaks down food small enough to drink — fiber and all.

We make a "nutriblast" every day with spinach, strawberries, blackberries, blueberries, peaches, flax seeds, pumpkin seeds, grapes, super green food powder, and either pomegranate juice and/or blueberry juice. The taste is amazing! It is pure nutrition. Cleanup is easy and takes about 30 seconds — unlike my old juicer with all of the leftover fiber mess. You can learn more about the NutriBullet at www.nutribullet.com.

Chapter 4   Supplements

Following our stated nutritional guidelines will give you an excellent foundation to prevent Alzheimer's. Adding certain nutritional supplements can give your body and brain additional support. Many doctors claim they if we simply eat right, we would not need nutritional supplements. Maybe that was true in the past, but with today's farming practices and depleted soils, we do not get the nutrition from our foods that previous generations did.

We begin by looking at supplements proven to help in preventing and delaying Alzheimer's. At the end of this chapter I will discuss cost and help you decide how to prioritize your supplements.

Everyone can benefit from a good quality multi-vitamin. However, choosing a multi-vitamin can be confusing. There are many different combinations of vitamins and minerals with a wide range of RDA percentages (recommended daily allowance). Think of the RDA as the minimum needed to prevent a vitamin deficiency disease (like scurvy or rickets), **not the amount you need for optimal health.**

My primary recommendation for a multivitamin is that it has a **high percentage of B complex**. It should state that on the front label. Be sure to look on the back label also, to see the actual percentage of the different B vitamins. I prefer one that has the RDA of the B vitamins in the 1,000% and up range. I realize this may sound like a lot. However, because it is water soluble, your body will use what it needs and excrete the rest. If you are under stress, you will need more of the B complex than the RDAs state for optimal health and well-being.

There are many types of multi-vitamins including natural, synthetic, wholefood, organic and those with or without minerals. I'm not going into the pros and cons of each one. *Livestrong.com*, as well as other sites have guides to help you make an informed choice.[1]

You will find a wide variety of costs between brands. Ideally everyone would get all of the best, highest quality, natural vitamins and supplements, but that can be very expensive. I would rather you take a cheaper synthetic vitamin than none at all. You will get at least some benefit from it. Get informed and make the choice that works for you.

Wal-mart has a line of low cost vitamins that can be purchased in store or on-line. You may also want to check out Vitacost.com and Puritan.com. value pricing. Most large chain drug stores have their own lower cost generic brand. You can also save money by using the store's loyalty card.

Acetyl-L-Carnitine

Acetyl-L-Carnitine is also known as **ALCAR.** ALCAR is an amino acid, a building block for proteins that helps the body produce energy. It works in the mitochondria, the "power plants" of all cells, boosting physical and mental energy.

ALCAR has been studied as a possible treatment for Alzheimer's disease, as it may have a protective effect on the brain and central nervous system. Experimental and clinical studies demonstrate that ALC may have a "**significant capacity to slow, and even reverse, the effects of aging on the brain,**" writes Dr. Russell L. Blaylock, in Health and Nutrition Secrets[2]

How does it work? ALCAR helps form the brain neurotransmitter, acetylcholine, which allows brain cells to pass along messages involving memory and learning. A lack of this neurotransmitter may be one of the causes of Alzheimer's. Many Alzheimer's drug therapies are based on this theory.

ALCAR helps regenerate neurons damaged by free radicals. Studies, involving old rats with memory loss, showed mitochondrial and oxidative damage to the DNA/RNA in their brains. The rats had ALCAR and **Alpha Lipoic Acid (ALA)** added to their drinking water. The results suggest that feeding ALCAR and ALA to old rats improves performance on memory tasks. The combination of ALCAR and LA worked best to reduce the effects of oxidation in the brain. When the hippocampus (one of the brain's memory centers) was studied by electron microscope, researchers found that **ALCAR and ALA reversed age-associated decay in the mitochondria.**[3]

Recommended daily dosage for acetyl-l-carnitine, ALCAR, is 500 mg/day and for alpha lipoic acid, ALA, it is 200 – 300 mg/day. ***When purchasing ALCAR, make sure the bottle says Acetyl-L-Carnitine, not just L-carnitine.**

Alpha Lipoic Acid

Alpha Lipoic Acid is considered one of the best antioxidants for protecting the brain. **Research shows that alpha lipoic acid may greatly reduce the progression of dementia.**[4] Livestrong.com reports the following about this nutrient:

> R-alpha lipoic acid is uniquely useful for providing antioxidant activity in brain cells because it is one of the few known antioxidants able to cross the blood-brain barrier.

> One of the hallmarks of Alzheimer's disease is the presence of plaques in your brain. Basically, plaques are clumps of protein that form during a reaction of excess metal ions that accumulate in your brain as you age. **As a strong metal chelator, R-alpha lipoic acid can bind to metal ions, leading researchers to believe it may be able to decrease the presence of plaques.** Although the mechanism is not entirely clear, experts **hypothesize R-alpha lipoic acid can reduce plaques in the brain by either inhibiting their formation or dissolving ones that already exist.**[5]

Recommended daily dosage for ALA (LA) is 200 – 300 mg/day.

Folic Acid

Folic acid is the man made version of folate, also called vitamin B-9. This water-soluble vitamin is part of the B complex. However, because it is water soluble, it is not stored in the fat and must be taken in daily. Folate is the form found in nature in many dark green vegetables, beans and citrus fruits. Folate/folic acid helps to form red blood cells and to synthesize and repair DNA.

Along with Vitamins B-12 and B-6, it helps the body clear excess homocysteine (explained in follow paragraphs) associated with cardiovascular disease and Alzheimer's. Folic acid appears to be neuroprotective and may help in the prevention of Alzheimer's disease. Following is a press release from *The National Institutes of Health (NIH) and The National Institute on Aging:*

Mouse experiments suggest that folic acid could play an essential role in protecting the brain against the ravages of Alzheimer's disease and other neurodegenerative disorders, according to scientists at the National Institute on Aging. This animal study could help researchers unravel the underlying biochemical mechanisms involved in another recent finding that concluded people with **high blood levels of homocysteine have nearly twice the risk of developing the disease.**

In the study, published in the March 1, 2002 issue of the *Journal of Neuroscience*, the investigators fed one group of mice with Alzheimer's-like plaques in their brains a diet that included normal amounts of folate while a second group was fed a diet deficient in this vitamin. These mice are transgenic, meaning they were bred with mutant genes that cause AD in people. They develop AD-like plaques in their brains that kill neurons.

The NIA team counted neurons in the hippocampus, a brain region critical for learning and memory that is destroyed as plaques accumulate during Alzheimer's disease. **The investigators found a decreased number of neurons in the mice fed the folic acid deficient diet.**

The scientists also discovered that mice with low amounts of dietary folic acid had elevated levels of homocysteine, an amino acid, in the blood and brain. They suspect that increased levels of homocysteine in the brain caused damage to the DNA of nerve cells in the hippocampus. In transgenic mice fed an adequate amount of folate, nerve cells in this brain region were able to repair damage to their DNA. But in the transgenic mice fed a folate-deficient diet, nerve cells were unable to repair this DNA damage.

These new findings establish a possible cause-effect relationship between elevated homocysteine levels and degeneration of nerve cells involved in learning and memory in a mouse model of Alzheimer's disease," said Mark Mattson, Ph.D., chief of the NIA's Laboratory of Neurosciences and the study's principal investigator.

People who have Alzheimer's disease often have low levels of folic acid in their blood, but it is not clear whether this is a result of the disease or if they are simply malnourished due to their illness. But based on emerging research, Dr. Mattson speculates consuming adequate amounts of folic acid — either in the diet or by supplementation — could be beneficial to the aging brain and help protect it against Alzheimer's and other neurodegenerative diseases.

Green leafy vegetables, citrus fruits and juices, whole wheat bread and dry beans are good sources of the vitamin. Since 1998, the Food and Drug Administration has required the addition of folic acid to enriched breads, cereals, flours, corn meals, pastas, rice, and other grain products. However, because it can take a long time for the symptoms of Alzheimer's disease to surface, researchers speculate it will be many years before folate supplementation in food could affect the incidence of dementia in the United States. A human clinical trial is being planned.[6]

In another study by Dutch scientists, folic acid was found to significantly improve the memory of older adults. Following is the report by *msnbc.msn.com*:

Taking large amounts of folic acid improved the memory of older adults, Dutch scientists reported Monday in the first study to show a vitamin pill might slow the mental decline of aging. The research adds to mounting evidence that a diet higher in folate — a B vitamin found in grains and certain dark-colored fruits and vegetables — is important for a variety of diseases. "As people age, some decline in brain function is inevitable. The Dutch study tested whether otherwise healthy people could slow that brain drain by taking double the recommended daily U.S. dose of folic acid — the amount in 2.5 pounds of strawberries.

The study divided 818 people ages 50 to 75 to take either a vitamin containing **800 micrograms of folic acid** a day, or a dummy pill, for three years. "**The folic acid protected users' brains**, lead researcher Jane Durga of Wageningen University reported Monday at a meeting of the Alzheimer's Association.

On memory tests, the supplement users had scores comparable to people 5.5 years younger, Durga said. On tests of cognitive speed, the folic acid helped users perform as well as people 1.9 years younger."

Another study in 2005 by scientists at the University of California, Irvine, found that men and women over age 60, **who regularly consumed at least 400 mcg. of folic acid through foods and supplements, cut their risk of developing Alzheimer's Disease by over 50%.**[7]

The recommended optimal daily dosage of folic acid is 800-1200 mcg. * Folic acid is most effective when taken with other B vitamin's (B complex) and especially with B-6 and B-12. More info is following on the combined synergies.

Vitamin B-12

B-12 is a water-soluble essential vitamin necessary for healthy functioning of the nervous system, the production of DNA and formation of red blood cells. Vitamin B-12 deficiency is common, especially among older people. Symptoms can include weakness, fatigue, shakiness, depression and poor memory. In fact, **severe vitamin B-12 deficiency can mimic the symptoms of Alzheimer's**. Research has shown that a vitamin B-12 deficiency will increase the risk of developing Alzheimer's. **However, large doses of B vitamins can cut the rate of brain shrinkage, as seen in Alzheimer's, by 50%.**[8]

Vitamin B-12 is naturally found only in animal products. It requires an acidic environment in the stomach to be digested. Many people do not have sufficient digestive acidity to absorb B-12. Stomach acid naturally decreases as we age.

Therefore, I recommend taking a high potency **sublingual** B-12. You simply put it under your tongue and let it dissolve. It will immediately be absorbed into the bloodstream via the sublingual artery. This is very similar to the B-12 shots often given for fatigue, but much less painful! Sublingual B-12 comes in several dosages. Minimal daily dosage should be 500 mcg. I take one that has 2500 mcg.

Vitamin B-6

Vitamin B6 (pyridoxine) is required for the body to make the neurotransmitters serotonin and norepinephrine, and for myelin formation. Myelin is the protective covering around nerves necessary for proper nerve transmission. Vitamin B-6 is found naturally in cereal grains, legumes, vegetables (carrots, spinach, peas), milk, cheese, eggs, fish, liver and meat. The recommended daily dosage of B-6 for homocysteine reduction is 50 mgs/day. **Vitamin B-6 is one of the trio of B vitamins that reduces dangerous excess homocysteine in the blood.**

Homocysteine Reduction

Homocysteine is an amino acid that can build up in the body and linked to numerous disease processes. **Homocysteine causes damage to the linings of arteries and other cells in the body.** Earlier in this chapter we discussed its link to Alzheimer's. Homocysteine also plays a role in cardiovascular disease, strokes, macular degeneration, hearing loss, some types of migraine, cancer and even depression.

Fortunately, homocysteine levels can be reduced in the body with the aid of three B vitamins — Folic Acid (B-9), B-6 and B-12. The combination of the three is key. **The three combined worked much better than taken individually.** They don't have to be in the same tablet or capsule, just taken near the same time. Numerous studies have been shown the relationship between these three B vitamins and homocysteine. Following is a report on the long running Nurse's Health Study:

In the ongoing Nurse's Health Study (*JAMA*, 2/4/98), researchers asked more than 80,000 women without heart disease about their diet and lifestyle at four times over 14 years. Those who had consumed more than 400 mcg of folate (folic acid) per day had the lowest risk of heart attack or dying of heart disease. Further, the lowest heart disease rates were found among those whose B6 intake was more than 3 mg a day.

Similarly, Omenn and colleagues (Circulation, 1998) measured the blood levels of folate, vitamin B6 and homocysteine in 800 healthy volunteers, and 750 people with vascular disease (e.g., stroke, coronary artery disease). They found that those with vascular disease had high homocysteine levels compared to the healthy volunteers. In men, high homocysteine was also significantly associated with low folate (folic acid) levels. Further, although many people with vascular disease did not have high homocysteine levels they often had low B6 levels. This latter finding suggests that low blood levels of B6 may contribute to heart disease even among those with normal homocysteine levels. [9]

Why is this important to Alzheimer's prevention?

According to *Wikipedia.org*, Vitamin B-12 deficiency may be associated with the onset and cause of Alzheimer's. Recent studies have found a relationship between B-12, homocysteine and Alzheimer's. A healthy brain must have "clean" free flowing blood vessels. Plaguing not only prevents needed nutrients from getting into the brain, but also increases the risk of stroke.

Vitamin D

Vitamin D is one of the most crucial nutrients our body requires. **In my opinion, it is the single most important vitamin to supplement.** The interesting thing about Vitamin D is that it naturally occurs in only a few foods. The obvious reason is that our bodies were designed to manufacture Vitamin D from the sun on our skin.

However, most of us spend the vast majority of our time inside and out of the sun. In the warmer months you would only need about 15 – 20 minutes, with arms and legs exposed, to get about **10,000 – 20,000 IUs** (international units) without sunscreen.

That's great for the summer, but what about the rest of the year? In the winter, if you live north of Atlanta, it is impossible to make vitamin D from sunlight because the sun never gets high enough in the sky for its ultraviolet B rays to penetrate the atmosphere.

Add to that, continually wearing sunscreen, and it is no wonder that so many people are deficient in this important vitamin. No one should get burned in the sun. That is not necessary to obtain maximum levels of vitamin D. However, constantly or frequently wearing sunscreen will block the skin from making vitamin D. Use common sense and don't get burned, but also allow enough time in the sun, without sunscreen, to let the body make an ample supply of this most valuable vitamin.

Vitamin D may have a key role in helping the brain to work well later in life, according to a study of 3000 European men between the ages of 40 and 79.

Vitamin D could be one of our body's main protections against damage from low levels of radiation, say radiological experts from the New York City Department of Health and

Mental Hygiene. Various studies have shown that people with adequate levels of vitamin D have a significantly lower risk of developing cancer, compared to people with lower levels. Vitamin D deficiency was found to be prevalent in cancer patients regardless of nutritional status, in a study carried out by Cancer Treatment Centers of America.[10]

What effect does Vitamin D have on preventing Alzheimer's? Let's look at one more study. This one is from *PsychCentral.com*:

Vitamin D3 may activate key genes and networks to help trigger the immune system to get rid of the amyloid beta protein, the core component of destructive plaques in the brain linked to Alzheimer's disease, according to a new study.

Previous lab work has shown that particular immune cells in people with Alzheimer's respond well to vitamin D3 and curcumin (found in turmeric spice) by stimulating the immune system to clear the brain of amyloid beta; however, researchers were unsure of exactly how this worked.

Vitamin D3 is the form that is produced by the skin with the help of sunlight and is also found in milk.

This new study helped clarify the key mechanisms involved, which will help us better understand the usefulness of vitamin D3 and curcumin as possible therapies for Alzheimer's disease," said study author Milan Fiala, M.D., a researcher at the David Geffen

School of Medicine at UCLA and the Veterans Affairs Greater Los Angeles Healthcare System.

Our findings demonstrate that active forms of vitamin D3 may be an important regulator of immune activities of macrophages in helping to clear amyloid plaques by directly regulating the expression of genes, as well as the structural physical workings of the cells," said study author Mizwicki, who was an assistant research biochemist in the department of biochemistry at UC Riverside when the study was conducted.[11]

In another study published in the Journal of Gerontology, researchers followed 489 women with an average age of 79.8. **After 7 years, the study found that the women who had the highest levels of Vitamin D, had the lowest risk — 77% less risk, of developing Alzheimer's disease.**[12]

What is a good daily dosage for maintaining health and lowering the risk of Alzheimer's? That's a good question. There is still much controversy over the recommended daily amount of Vitamin D.

Many experts knowledgeable in optimal dosages agree that 5,000 IUs daily is a good minimal amount. To be more exact, have your blood levels checked and begin by taking 1,000 IU per 25 pounds of body weight. A person who weighs 150 pounds, for instance, would take 6,000 IU per day as a starting dose. Ideally, your blood level should be around 60-80 ng/ml, as this allows the body to have some vitamin D in reserve, and it duplicates the higher levels found in young, healthy individuals who spend a decent amount of time in the sun.[13]

I personally take 10,000-20,000 per day, about the same amount received from spending 15-20 minutes in the sun. If you have medium to dark skin tone, then longer time in the sun is required to get the same amount of Vitamin D. Also, if you are obese, you will not make nearly as much Vitamin D when in the sun.

Taking magnesium can help. **Vitamin D is better assimilated in the presence of sufficient magnesium, which helps open cell membrane receptor sites. I recommend taking magnesium citrate** because it is better absorbed than other forms. It usually comes in a powder. Mix with water and drink, along with your Vitamin D supplements.

The wonderful thing about magnesium is that it is a natural muscle relaxer and helps calm the nervous system. Many people feel better and sleep better when taking magnesium citrate. Start with about ¼ teaspoon mixed in a glass of water. Each day you can increase the amount until you begin to have looser stools. Back off slightly from that amount and you will have your personal maximum daily amount.

Krill Oil and Omega 3's

Omega 3's essential fatty acids are part of the "good fats" we mentioned earlier. One of the newer supplements is krill oil, made from small sea creatures similar to shrimp. **The great thing about krill oil is that it contains very concentrated omega 3's.** If you were used to taking large fish oil supplements for your omega 3's, you can now get the same amount in a much smaller soft gel. Following is an excellent article from the web site *Heart-health-for-life.com*.

Krill oil benefits seem too good to be true... but not when you realize that they affect every cell in your body! Fats and oils expert Udo Erasmus, PhD, author of *Fats That Kill and Fats That Heal* says, "**95% of the population is deficient in omega 3 oils.**"

If you've had trouble remembering things lately, maybe it's time to "oil up" your brain and heart arteries. One of the best brain nutrients is krill oil, the most powerful omega 3 oil on the planet. In his book, The Perricone Prescription, Dr. Nicholas Perricone explains how it works. "Brain function is intimately tied to our essential fatty acid intake. Omega 3 fatty acids make up the phospholipid bilayer of the cell membrane which is critical in the proper functioning of the nerve cells of to our brains."

Our brains are 60% fat and ideally one-third of this should be omega 3 oils. It gets a little technical here but stay with me. Look at it as a "workout" for your brain. Essential fatty acids, also called EFAs, are called Essential because your body cannot get along without them. These fats, which are known as omega 3 oils, have long unpronounceable names and are known by the initials **DHA, EPA and ALA**.

When plaque builds up on arterial walls and then breaks loose, it forms a clot. If this clot restricts an artery in the brain, it causes a stroke and when it occurs in a heart artery it results in a heart attack. Research shows that the Omega 3 DHA helps dissolve clots before they can cause any damage.

Heart health and brain health go together like apple pie and ice cream. DHA and EPA are found in fish oil and in great abundance in Krill Oil. ALA is found in nuts and flax seed. DHA provides one of the greatest benefits to the heart and brain.

If the oil in your body is laden with sludge-like chemically modified Omega 6 vegetable oils, the signals to and from your brain get through slowly...or not at all. Krill oil provides the perfect medium to accelerate the movement of information to and from your brain.

Now, UCLA scientists have confirmed that the omega 3 oils in fish and krill oil can help prevent

Alzheimer's disease, and they have identified the reasons why.

Greg Cole, professor of medicine and neurology at the David Geffen School of Medicine, and his team of researchers, have discovered that the **omega-3 fatty acid (DHA) found in krill and fish oils increased the production of a protein which is known to destroy the "plaques" that form in the brains of Alzheimer's victims.**

Other benefits of krill oil are:

It is 5 times more bioavailable than fish oil which means that you can use far less and get more omega 3 benefits. Since it is harvested from the icy waters of the Antarctica you have no worries about dangerous heavy metals or contaminants that may be found in fish and some fish oils. Krill oil contains one of the most powerful inflammation fighters ever discovered. It's highly concentrated omega-3s turn off excess inflammation like a switch.[14]

How much daily krill oil to take? It depends on the brand. If you compare brands, you will find some have more of the omega 3's of EPA and DHA than others per 300 mg. soft gel. Therefore, 1-3 soft gels per day is a good amount.

DHA

DHA, as mentioned above, is an **Omega 3 essential fatty acid. It may be the most**

important one for the brain. The following article could have also gone in the nutrition chapter. It explains why we need to decrease the amount of fructose in our diet. I'm adding it in here at this point because it also tells about a new finding involving DHA and fructose. The article is a little long, but very interesting and informative. It is from the UCLA newsroom:

Attention, college students cramming between midterms and finals: Binging on soda and sweets for as little as six weeks may make you stupid.

A new UCLA rat study is the first to show how a diet steadily high in fructose slows the brain, hampering memory and learning — and how omega-3 fatty acids can counteract the disruption. The peer-reviewed Journal of Physiology publishes the findings in its May 15 edition.

Our findings illustrate that what you eat affects how you think," said Fernando Gomez-Pinilla, a professor of neurosurgery at the David Geffen School of Medicine at UCLA and a professor of integrative biology and physiology in the UCLA College of Letters and Science. "Eating **a high-fructose diet over the long term alters your brain's ability to learn and remember information. But adding omega-3 fatty acids to your meals can help minimize the damage.**"

While earlier research has revealed how fructose harms the body through its role in diabetes, obesity and fatty liver, this study is the first to uncover how the sweetener influences the brain.

Sources of fructose in the Western diet include cane sugar (sucrose) and high-fructose corn syrup, an inexpensive liquid sweetener. The syrup is widely added to processed foods, including soft drinks, condiments, applesauce and baby food. The average American consumes roughly 47 pounds of cane sugar and 35 pounds of high-fructose corn syrup per year, according to the U.S. Department of Agriculture.

We're less concerned about naturally occurring fructose in fruits, which also contain important antioxidants," explained Gomez-Pinilla, who is also a member of UCLA's Brain Research Institute and Brain Injury Research Center. "We're more concerned about the fructose in high-fructose corn syrup, which is added to manufactured food products as a sweetener and preservative."

Gomez-Pinilla and study co-author Rahul Agrawal, a UCLA visiting postdoctoral fellow from India, studied two groups of rats that each consumed a fructose solution as drinking water for six weeks. The second group also received omega-3 fatty acids in the form of flaxseed oil and docosahexaenoic acid (DHA), which protects against damage to the synapses — the chemical connections between brain cells that enable memory and learning.

DHA is essential for synaptic function — brain cells' ability to transmit signals to one another," Gomez-Pinilla said. "This is the mechanism that makes learning and memory possible. **Our bodies can't produce enough DHA, so it must be supplemented through our diet."**

The animals were fed standard rat chow and trained on a maze twice daily for five days before starting the experimental diet. The UCLA team tested how well the rats were able to navigate the maze, which contained numerous holes but only one exit. The scientists placed visual landmarks in the maze to help the rats learn and remember the way.

"Six weeks later, the researchers tested the rats' ability to recall the route and escape the maze. What they saw surprised them.

The second group of rats navigated the maze much faster than the rats that did not receive omega-3 fatty acids," Gomez-Pinilla said. "The DHA-deprived animals were slower, and their brains showed a decline in synaptic activity. Their brain cells had trouble signaling each other, disrupting the rats' ability to think clearly and recall the route they'd learned six weeks earlier."

The DHA-deprived rats also developed signs of resistance to insulin, a hormone that controls blood sugar and regulates synaptic function in the brain. **A closer look at the rats' brain tissue suggested that insulin had lost much of its power to influence the brain cells**.

Because insulin can penetrate the blood–brain barrier, the hormone may signal neurons to trigger reactions that disrupt learning and cause memory loss," Gomez-Pinilla said.

He suspects that fructose is the culprit behind the DHA-deficient rats' brain dysfunction. Eating too much fructose could block insulin's ability to regulate how cells use and store sugar for the energy required for processing thoughts and emotions.

Insulin is important in the body for controlling blood sugar, but it may play a different role in the brain, where insulin appears to disturb memory and learning," he said. "Our study shows that a high-fructose diet harms the brain as well as the body. This is something new."

Gomez-Pinilla, a native of Chile and an exercise enthusiast who practices what he preaches, advises people to keep fructose intake to a minimum and swap sugary desserts for fresh berries and Greek yogurt, which he keeps within arm's reach in a small refrigerator in his office. An occasional bar of dark chocolate that hasn't been processed with a lot of extra sweetener is fine too, he said.

Still planning to throw caution to the wind and indulge in a hot-fudge sundae? Then also eat foods rich in omega-3 fatty acids, like salmon, walnuts and flaxseeds, or take a daily DHA capsule. Gomez-Pinilla recommends one gram (1,000 mg) of DHA per day.

Our findings suggest that consuming DHA regularly protects the brain against fructose's harmful effects," said Gomez-Pinilla. "It's like saving money in the bank. You want to build a reserve for your brain to tap when it requires extra fuel to fight off future diseases.[15]

You can buy DHA separately or take DHA and krill oil together for optimal protection. Daily dosage recommendations for DHA are 800-1000 mg/day. (1000mg = 1 gram).

Aspirin, Advil and Aleve

To help prevent heart attacks, many people are advised by their medical doctors to take a baby aspirin each day (81mg). **Obviously, this isn't for everyone**. There may be side effects, such as intestinal bleeding, and interactions with other medications. If you have questions concerning whether this is right for you, please check with your medical doctor.

Aspirin can help in prevention of cardiovascular problems because it lowers the overall amount of inflammation in the body. It also helps prevent platelet clumping in the blood, allowing for less potential plaguing and better blood flow.

But, what about using anti-inflammatories such as aspirin, Advil or Aleve for prevention of Alzheimer's? **Inflammation is believed to be a contributor to the development of the disease.**

Following is part of an interview with *CNN's* medical correspondent, Dr. Sanjay Gupta, discussing the possible benefits and risks of aspirin therapy, with *CNN* anchor Bill Hemmer:

GUPTA: I recommend [aspirin] to a lot of my patients for all sorts of things. Thinning the blood, preventing stroke, heart attacks, possibly reducing the risk of colon cancer and now, as you say, Bill, possibly also preventing Alzheimer's disease.

This isn't brand new stuff, but it's starting to become more and more obvious. They looked at more than 3,000 people in Utah, people who were either near dementia or actually developed signs of dementia — early signs of Alzheimer's disease — and they looked at what their use of nonsteroidal anti-inflammatory medications are.

That is like Ibuprofen, Advil or aspirin, and they found that people who actually took those medications long term — that is longer than two years, four times a week — actually had a 45 percent risk reduction of Alzheimer's disease.

HEMMER: As it relates to Alzheimer's, how does this work within the body?

GUPTA: Let me just say first of all that not everyone is on board with this. There are some risks to taking these medications. This isn't a medication that people necessarily want to go out and start taking right away. There is some risk of gastrointestinal bleeding.

But there are a couple of theories. **One is that Alzheimer's disease is caused by an inflammatory process in the brain. Simply put, if you take an anti-inflammatory, you might reduce the risk of Alzheimer's.**

There is another theory about this as well. When you have Alzheimer's disease, you have a couple of enzymes in the brain that cause a breakdown of a couple of proteins. Eventually when that protein is split, it forms something called amyloid plaque.

The name is not important, but imagine plaques of material in the brain disrupting some activity when it comes to neuronal transmission, things like that, possibly even leading to cell death. Anti-inflammatory medications are supposed to break that process down, not let it occur.

HEMMER: I can see some people ... saying, "I need to start taking aspirin, if indeed I am getting up into that age — 55, 60, 65." Is that recommended?

GUPTA: I think that it may be coming when you have a strong family history, or if somebody in your family has had Alzheimer's before. They may say, "Listen, you have no signs of dementia; you have no problems at all. Maybe a little memory loss like everyone does from time to time. But start taking your aspirin now so that you will have it in place; you will have the anti-inflammatory mechanisms in place, to stave off the Alzheimer's later on.[16]

One important note I found when looking at the aspirin/Alzheimer's prevention research is **that aspirin (or Advil or Aleve) worked best in those who had NO obvious signs yet of Alzheimer's. It did not help any in people who already had definite symptoms of dementia.**

Other supplements

This is not a complete list of all potentially effective supplements for Alzheimer's prevention. There are other supplements that may have a beneficial effect on the brain and our aging bodies. However, I believe the ones listed in this chapter have the most conclusive research, at this time, to support them.

I realize cost of supplements is a consideration for many people. I want to give you an idea of approximate costs to begin taking what I have recommended, using lower cost vitamins. **If you are starting from scratch and use a low cost supplier, you would probably spend about $ 85.00 (plus S&H) to get started.** If you can afford to buy both larger quantities of bottles and larger bottles (more pills per bottle) you can receive substantial savings.

Average cost of individual supplements (one month supply only) from low cost online provider:

Multi-vitamin with high B complex —$ 12.99

Vitamin D (D3) — $3.95

Magnesium Citrate — $ 7.79

Folic Acid — $ 3.99

Sublingual B-12 — $ 5.95

Acetyl-l-carnitine — $ 6.95

Alpha Lipoic Acid (ALA) — $ 6.95

Krill Oil — $15.99

Aspirin — $ 5.95

DHA — $ 12.99

Total — $83.50

If cost is a consideration, then start at the top of this list and work down. If necessary, you can cut costs by not taking every supplement every day. It's OK to spread them out a little bit.

Another idea is to go in together with friends or family and order in bulk. Several companies have offers of buy 3, get 2 free, or free shipping and handling with a certain dollar amount order.

Chapter 5   Physical Exercise

Physical exercise is one of the best ways to protect your brain. It increases blood flow and delivers much needed oxygen. We shouldn't be surprised that exercise also helps keep the brain from deteriorating and is one of the best ways to prevent Alzheimer's. In a research brief posted on the *alzforum.org*. web site, we find the following:

> Although a growing number of studies suggest that exercise can keep an aging brain honed and perhaps ward off dementia, only a couple of those studies have included objective measures of activity.

> To better quantify the effect of exercise, researchers led by Aron Buchman at Rush University, Chicago, Illinois, measured total daily activity in more than 700 healthy seniors, average age 82, who participated in the Rush Memory and Aging Project. The volunteers wore an actigraph device, which records all movements, on their wrists around the clock for about nine days. In the April 24 Neurology, the authors report that **participants with the highest levels of total daily activity had a slower rate of cognitive decline and about half the risk of developing Alzheimer's disease over the next four years than the least active participants.**[1]

Physical exercise appears to have greater impact on maintaining healthy brain function than any other aspect studied. Livestrong.com. gave this report:

Studies exploring the relationship between aerobic exercise and brain health have produced some startling findings that are expected to have profound implications for future treatments of a wide range of conditions. **Research suggests that exercise is the trigger that sets in motion the brain's capacity to self-correct various deficiencies, including those caused by age-related cognitive decline, alcoholism and radiation therapy.**

A long-term study of 1,449 people aged 65 to 79, conducted at Stockholm's Karolinska Institute, found that **those who had exercised at least twice a week in middle age were 50 percent less likely to develop dementia and 60 percent less likely to develop Alzheimer's disease in old age.** The study, published in the October 4, 2005, online edition of *The Lancet Neurology*, noted that **even participants genetically predisposed to Alzheimer's, who had a history of regular aerobic exercise, were at reduced risk of developing the devastating brain disease.**[2]

Angela Lunde of the *Mayo Clinic* wrote the following in her blog:

Mounting evidence suggests that physical activity may have benefits beyond a healthy heart and body weight. Through the past several years, **population studies have suggested that exercise which raises your heart rate for at least 30 minutes several times a week can lower your risk of Alzheimer's. Physical activity appears to inhibit Alzheimer's-like brain changes in mice, slowing the development of a key feature of the disease.**

In one observational study, investigators looked at the relationship of physical activity and mental function in about 6,000 women age 65 and older, over an 8 year period. They found that the women who were more physically active were less likely to experience a decline in their mental function than inactive women.

Another compelling study, conducted by researchers at the University of Chicago, was highlighted on *ABC News*. The study used mice bred to develop Alzheimer's type plaque in the brain. In the study, some mice were allowed to exercise and others were not. **The brains in the physically active mice had 50 to 80 percent less plaque than the brains of the sedentary mice and they (exercising mice) produced significantly more of an enzyme in the brain that <u>prevents</u> plaque.**

Dr. Ronald Petersen, director of the Alzheimer's Research Center at the Mayo Clinic, said on *ABC*: "Regular physical exercise is probably the best means we have of preventing Alzheimer's disease today, better than medications, better than intellectual activity, better than supplements and diet.[3]

Further evidence comes from the *Livestrong.com* web site:

A lack of exercise affects Alzheimer's disease in a profound way. The link between exercise and Alzheimer's became more and more clear between the years from 2008 to 2011. There is a growing body of evidence that aerobic exercise slows the mental decline of people who have Alzheimer's. Beyond those findings, there is a growing body of evidence indicating that regular exercise may prevent or delay the symptoms of

Alzheimer's. The Alzheimer's Association predicted that 10 million baby boomers in America will develop the disease. Those are frightening statistics, so if you fall into that age group, you might want to get out there and work out. Exercise is proven to be good for your heart and it appears to be good for your brain as well.

The New York Times reported that exercise seemed to lower the risk for Alzheimer's disease, as did eating a healthy, Mediterranean type of diet. In a major study at Columbia University, 1,880 people in their seventies were followed and assessed in terms of their level of physical activity, diet and incidence of Alzheimer's. During the five years of the study, 282 cases of the disease were diagnosed. The people with the healthiest diets were 40 percent less likely to develop the disease than those who ate the worst diets. People who exercised the most were 37 percent less likely to contract Alzheimer's as people who didn't exercise at all. **If you were in the top third for best diet and most exercise, your chances of being diagnosed with Alzheimer's were 59 percent less than people in the bottom third.**

Another link between exercise and its ability to prevent Alzheimer's was established in a study from Washington University in St. Louis. Published in the September issue of *Annals of Neurology*, and reported by the *Alzheimer's Reading Room* website, the study of 69 people from ages 55 to 88 measured the association between exercise and Alzheimer's biomarkers, levels of proteins in the brain characteristic of the disease. The more people exercised, the fewer biomarkers were detected. One of the researchers, Denise Head, concluded, "It may be useful for physicians to recommend exercise engagement, not only for

Alzheimer's symptoms but also potentially for preventive care."

A Seattle study published in the *Archives of Neurology* in January 2011 concluded that regular aerobic exercise could protect and even reverse mild cognitive impairment, which are early signs of Alzheimer's. A group of 33 men and women with mild cognitive impairment were divided into an aerobic exercise group that rode a stationary bike or walked on a treadmill for 45 to 60 minutes four times per week, and a control group that did stretching and balancing exercises. **After six months, the aerobic group displayed significant advances in mental agility, while the control group continued their decline in thinking speed, word fluency and ability to multi-task.** The Seattle study is considered one of the first to show that exercise can protect the human brain and perhaps ward off or even reverse symptoms of Alzheimer's. The tentative link established in 2008 became a well-supported theory in 2011, a great advance in Alzheimer's research in just four years.[4]

We've seen many types of exercise that protect the brain and help prevent Alzheimer's. But, does one type of exercise provide a better benefit than others? Possibly. This summary from *CNN.com* highlights the differences:

It's well-known that exercising to maintain a healthy heart also helps create a healthy mind. But several new studies suggest that when it comes to preventing dementia, not all forms of exercise are created equal.

Studies presented at this year's Alzheimer's Association International Conference found that **resistance training was particularly beneficial for improving the cognitive abilities of older adults.**

While the studies were small, all including 150 participants or less, they did seem to indicate that resistance training — such as weight lifting or using resistance bands — could possibly be an intervention for dementia in older adults.

One study divided a group of 86 women, all between the ages of 70 and 80, into three different exercise groups: Weight lifting, walking, or balance and tone exercises. Each group did the exercises twice a week for 6 months. Everyone appeared to benefit from the exercise.

We actually imaged their brains, using functional MRIs — and these people showed better brain function," explained lead investigator, Dr. Teresa Liu Ambrose.

Participants were tested for cognitive executive functions such as attention, memory and planning. According to Ambrose, "the cognitive executive function and associated memory — those are the two traits most linked to dementia."

At the end of the trial, those in the weight lifting group were most improved.[5]

The **hippocampus** is a region of the brain where memories are stored, indexed and organized. It is activated in the process of learning. **Science has shown the volume of**

the hippocampus decreases by about 1-2%
per year beginning around age 30. In
Alzheimer's disease, the hippocampus is one
of the first areas in the brain, to be affected.

But, there is good news. **Exercise not only
prevents the normal shrinkage (atrophy)
from occurring, but also stimulates
neurogenesis — the formation of new brain
cells and connections! So, not only can you
keep your brain from shrinking, but you can
make it even bigger and stronger.** Various
studies have shown benefits from exercise.
Walking, running and weight training all
improve brain function. The following article
from Cellmedicine.com further explains this
process:

It has always been understood, at least intuitively if
not scientifically, that physical exercise is important for
proper health, mentally as well as physically. Indeed, a
number of previous studies have indicated that people
who engage in regular physical exercise score higher on
memory tests than people who do not exercise. Now,
researchers at Columbia University have shed some
light on the specific mechanisms that are at work in the
mental benefits that result from physical exercise.

Physical exercise targets a region within the
hippocampus that is known as the dentate gyrus, a
specialized region of the brain which is involved in
memory, among other neurological processes. When the
neurons of the dentate gyrus begin to atrophy over the

years, the person is said to suffer age-related memory decline. **Conversely, the growth of new neurons within the dentate gyrus will prevent memory decline – and this is exactly what happens as a result of physical exercise.** Using MRI (magnetic resonance imaging), the researchers at Columbia University have now revealed that **neurogenesis (the growth of new neurons) is stimulated in the dentate gyrus region immediately following physical exercise. These new nerve cells provide protection against the loss of memory with age.**

In the past, prior to MRI technology, neurogenesis was observable only via postmortem examination, from which it was found that **age-related memory decline typically begins around 30 years of age.** However, the onset of memory decline was associated with this age only because this has traditionally been the stage of life at which people tend to become more habitually sedentary in their lifestyles, and less inclined toward serious physical exercise. **By contrast, by prolonging regular physical exercise throughout life, neurogenesis in the dentate gyrus can continue up to any age.**[6]

Get moving! Head to the gym, the biking path, walking trails or the pool. Get those weights or resistive bands out of the closet and put them to work. Run, dance, ski, skate, row, hula hoop – anything that gets your heart rate up for at least 30 minutes and builds strong muscles. You will protect your brain, save your memory and prevent Alzheimer's!

Chapter 6   Cognitive Reserve and Brain Training

Cognitive reserve describes the brain's ability to function **even when physical pathology and deterioration is present.** The really good news is that cognitive reserve can be built up. It's like adding money to a savings account for a rainy day.

One of the factors contributing to cognitive reserve is higher education. If you went to college and obtained a degree, then you already have an edge in preventing Alzheimer's. The following article from *alzinfo.org* explains in more detail:

Education may provide mental reserves that help to keep the brain agile into old age. Those are the findings of a new study from researchers at Washington University School of Medicine in St. Louis.

Other studies have shown similar correlations between years of education and risk of Alzheimer's disease. **But the current study suggested that even those individuals whose brains appeared "scarred" by Alzheimer's could still be cognitively normal, especially if they had received more years of formal education.**

The researchers found that seniors with the most years of formal education scored higher on tests of memory, learning and thinking compared to those who spent the least time in school. In fact, many of the highly educated individuals who did well on the memory tests were shown by imaging tests to have the same kind of damage seen in the brains of those with Alzheimer's disease. The findings were published in the *Archives of Neurology*, one of the medical journals from the *American Medical Association*.

The findings support the cognitive reserve theory, which refers to the brain's ability to nurture healthy brain cells and connections between them. As people age, diseases like Alzheimer's ravage the brain with the buildup of toxic proteins that form plaques and tangles. But according to the cognitive reserve theory, if enough healthy brain cells and brain cell connections remain, people can escape symptoms like memory loss and disordered thinking that are typical of Alzheimer's disease.

Education is thought to boost cognitive reserve. Intellectual challenges to the brain early in life from schoolwork are thought to build brain cells and enrich the connections between them, effects that may be maintained into later years.

Earlier studies of normal aging have found that higher levels of educational attainment were associated with less cognitive and functional decline. And having few years of formal education has also been linked to an increased risk of Alzheimer's. A study last year from Finland found, for example, that teenage dropouts were at higher risk of developing Alzheimer's years later than those who got their diplomas and continued with further study.

Intellectually stimulating careers and hobbies, like learning a new language, playing a musical instrument or doing crossword puzzles or word games, build extra brainpower. Healthier brain cells and connections may help compensate for the rise in Alzheimer's-like brain changes that accompany normal aging.

In the study, Catherine M. Roe, Ph.D., and colleagues at Washington University studied nearly 200 seniors (mean age 67) over a five-year period. Thirty-seven had a diagnosis of Alzheimer's disease, while 161 had no signs of dementia.

The researchers injected the study participants with a radioactive substance called Pittsburgh compound B, and then scanned their brains using an advanced imaging technique called positron emission tomography, or PET. The imaging agent, developed by scientists at the University of Pittsburgh Medical Center, indicates brain areas damaged by Alzheimer's by attaching to deposits of beta-amyloid, the toxic protein that builds up and forms plaques in the brains of those with the disease.

In the study, certain individuals' brains absorbed the most Pittsburgh compound B, an indication that their brains were riddled with the greatest numbers of beta-amyloid plaques. But the more years of education that they had, the less likely they were to perform poorly on memory and thinking tests. In other words, their education seemed to protect them against the memory loss and other symptoms of Alzheimer's disease.

The results support the hypothesis that cognitive reserve influences the association between Alzheimer's disease pathological burden and cognition," the authors wrote.

It is thought that symptoms of Alzheimer's would eventually emerge as beta-amyloid plaques continue to accumulate, even in the most highly educated people. **But for many seniors, living into their 70s and 80s sharp as a tack, education and mental stimulation is thought to strengthen cognitive reserve and possibly protect against Alzheimer's. And many people will die of other causes before the effects of Alzheimer's become evident.**[1]

If you have a college degree, you may already have some cognitive reserve. But, is it enough to keep you from developing Alzheimer's? And, what if you dropped out of school or never got that college degree? Is it too late for you? **Not unless you already have moderate to significant mental decline.** If you can follow the contents of this book and remember at least some of the primary points, then you can still likely build cognitive reserve.

When I ask people what they know about preventing Alzheimer's, most reply to do crossword puzzles and read. Crossword puzzles are good, if you enjoy them and do them often. Doing one occasionally is not enough to help. That's like exercising once a week. Both physical and mental exercise must be done **several times a week, at a certain intensity,** to be of benefit. If it doesn't **challenge you,** it will not build and maintain important new neural connections.

Casual walking doesn't do much to prevent Alzheimer's, although it is a better choice than sitting home watching TV. But, if you step it up, walk faster, go up and down hills and a further distance, then you will achieve real benefit.

The same principle holds true for your brain. You must do more than read novels for enjoyment. While that is helpful for stress relief, which we cover in the next chapter, it will not build cognitive reserve to prevent Alzheimer's.

You must challenge your brain, as in memory recall, learning or doing something new. Crossword puzzles are good, if they challenge you. I've never been good at crosswords. They often ask questions about topics that don't interest me, so I don't do them.

However, my daughter turned me on to Sudoku. It's a bit like a crossword puzzle, but using numbers. There is a grid of nine blocks across and nine down. Within the large grid are smaller grids of three blocks across and three down. The goal of the puzzle seems so simple. Just use each number 1- 9 one time only on each line, across, down and within each mini-block.

It always starts out easy and then traps you as you get into corners or have most of the puzzle filled in. Then, you have to go back and re-do lines until you can make it all work out. I'm still working on the "easy" categories. That's OK. The point is to make your brain work. It doesn't matter if you actually finish the puzzle or not — even though it does give you a sense of satisfaction.

It's easy to get into a comfortable rut. Come home from work, fix yummy comfort food for dinner, relax on sofa, get sleepy and go to bed. I know young working moms are thinking, "I wish!" You may be chasing kids around, helping them with baths and homework, trying to do housework and prepare dinner, all at the same time. That's actually much better for your brain in the long run.

We tend to slow down after the children grow up. As we age, our hormones change and energy lags. Stress and responsibilities of life overwhelm many, leading to depression. They're more concerned about surviving the moment than planning for the future. I understand. I've been there. But, at some point, you must determine a plan for your life and begin to work that plan.

With no children at home, I now have more time to work on myself. I decided to take up French again. I took French classes in school from the 4th grade thru college. I lacked one class being able to graduate and was able to KLEP an intermediate French course. I read French but was slow in speaking and comprehending native speakers. I wanted to be fluent.

Many years have passed and I never had a reason to speak French. I know it is buried down deep in the recesses of my brain, but it will take some work to bring it out.

I thought I would try the Rosetta Stone French series. But, it's a bit expensive. I found some conversational French CDs for $10.00 and a used French text book. I love it! You don't have to spend a lot of money to make progress. Be creative. That's good for your brain, too.

My goal is to become fluent. Once I've conquered French, then I will start on Spanish. Who knows after that? Maybe Chinese...or maybe, not. I'll just stick to the easier Romance languages. My goal is to continually learn and be challenged. If you stop learning, you've given up. Find what's interesting to you, master it and move on to the next challenge.

Research has shown that learning a new language is one of the best ways to build cognitive reserve. The following article from *Psychcental.com* explains:

Speaking more than one language can not only make travel less of a hassle — it may also enhance mental health. Investigators combined behavioral research with neuroimaging technology to determine the effect of bilingualism on cognitive skills and as protection from symptoms of dementia. The research raises the possibility that increasing diversity in world populations may have an unexpected positive impact on the resiliency of the adult brain.

Previous studies have established that bilingualism has a beneficial effect on cognitive development in children," said lead study author Ellen Bialystok, a Distinguished Research Professor of Psychology at York University in Toronto. "In our paper, we reviewed recent studies using both behavioral and neuroimaging methods to examine the effects of bilingualism on cognition in adults."

In the study, researchers discuss the intriguing finding that as an individual monitors two languages — in a quest to determine which language is more appropriate — brain regions are activated that pertain to general attention and cognitive control.

Researchers believe use of the cognitive control networks for bilingual language processing may reconfigure and strengthen them. The internal exercise may enhance "mental flexibility," the ability to adapt to ongoing changes and process information efficiently.

Researchers say that the studies also suggest that **bilingualism improves "cognitive reserve," the protective effect that stimulating mental or physical activity has on cognitive functioning in healthy aging.**

Cognitive reserve is believed to slow the onset of symptoms in those suffering from dementia. **This premise is supported by studies showing that bilinguals experience onset symptoms of dementia years later than monolinguals.**

Our conclusion is that lifelong experience in managing attention to two languages reorganizes specific brain networks, creating a more effective basis for executive control and sustaining better cognitive performance throughout the lifespan, said Bialystok.[2]

Playing a musical instrument also builds cognitive reserve. If you have an old musical instrument in the closet, pull it out and start practicing again. If you never played an instrument, but think you would like to, then it's not too late. Often a friend or family member has an instrument that you could use. They can help you get started.

Another idea is to look at yard sales. Musical instruments are often found for a "song". Look online at Youtube.com and other sites for free instruction. The following article from *Philly.com* is an excellent piece about the mental benefits of playing a musical instrument.

A growing body of evidence suggests that learning to play an instrument and continuing to practice and play it may offer mental benefits throughout life. Hearing has also been shown to be positively affected by making music.

The latest study, published in the July issue of *Frontiers in Human Neuroscience*, shows that **musical instrument training may reduce the effects of mental decline associated with aging**. The research found that older adults who learned music in childhood and continued to play an instrument for at least 10 years outperformed others in tests of memory and cognitive ability.

It also revealed that sustaining musical activity during advanced age may enhance thinking ability, neutralizing any negative impact of age and even lack of education. It's unclear; however, whether starting an instrument in adulthood provides any mental advantages.

"Behaviors can change your brain," said study author Brenda Hanna-Pladdy, an assistant professor of neurology, radiology and imaging sciences at Emory University, in Atlanta.

The study confirms and refines findings from previous research published April 2011 in the journal Neuropsychology.

In childhood, when the brain is still developing, it seems that learning a musical instrument and continuing to play it for at least a decade or more may lay the groundwork for benefits later in life, Hanna-Pladdy said. But it's also valuable to then pick up the instrument in middle age and start playing again, she noted.

In this study, 70 musicians and non-musicians aged 59 to 80 were evaluated by neuropsychological tests and surveyed about general lifestyle activities. **The musicians scored higher on tests of mental acuity, visual-spatial judgment, verbal memory and recall, and motor dexterity.**

Why study music education as opposed to calculus or history? One reason is that evaluating the impact of music education is relatively easy because most people can specifically quantify the number of years they studied an instrument, Hanna-Pladdy said. It's also simpler to quantify the time spent playing music than hours devoted to other activities, such as crossword puzzles, reading or playing games. "Musical activity requires years of practice and is a challenging cognitive exercise," she said.

Cheryl Grady, a senior scientist at the Rotman Research Institute at Baycrest Centre, in Toronto, said the research confirms what has been known for some time: Education can help protect against cognitive decline in older adults.

She has studied the impact of learning a second language on the brain, which Grady said is related to the need to inhibit one language system when speaking, reading or thinking in the other. **The mental process required to play a musical instrument may work in the same way as juggling dual languages to strengthen the connections in your brain over time**, she noted.[3]

We've looked at crossword puzzles, Sudoku, learning a new language, and playing a musical instrument as ways to improve cognitive reserve and prevent Alzheimer's. What else can you do? Anything that challenges your mind and is enjoyable, so that you will continue to do it over time.

For example, take sewing or quilting. There are so many beautiful patterns to choose from. You can quilt by hand or machine. Piecing patterns together requires hand-eye coordination and makes your brain work harder. That's what we want. Woodworking is similar.

Let's go back to reading again. Casual reading doesn't build cognitive reserve. On the other hand, reading to learn new facts, stimulates your brain to build new neural pathways. Time spent mentally reviewing facts recently learned, can take a short term memory, send it to long term memory and build cognitive reserve.

Brain training is a fast growing industry. Many web sites now offer personalized training programs designed to improve cognitive reserve, memory and recall. I personally use the web site *Lumosity.com*.

The program tracks your training and exercise scores. One such score is called the BPI (Brain Performance Index). It measures cognitive performance based on the combined results of your best games in each Brain Area — Memory, Attention, Speed, Flexibility and Problem Solving. According to Luminosity.com., on average, BPI increases 50% after playing 100 games. That's impressive. *Lumosity.com* is a paid web site. One year costs $79. Discounts are available for multiple years and a free trial period is offered. If you don't want to commit to a paid site, look for free web sites that offer brain games.

One obvious way to challenge the memory is with— wait for it — **memorization**. I hear you groaning already. Maybe memorizing brings back bad memories of "cramming" for college exams. The problem with "cramming" is that we memorize facts to pass a test, knowing we will never need to recall that fact again. Therefore, the facts learned never make it to long term memory. There are techniques you can use while memorizing that will automatically develop more neural connections, making it easier to recall. Entire books have been written about these processes, so I will not elaborate here. Googling the words "memory" or "improve memory" will give you additional information.

What would you be interested in memorizing? Before you say, "nothing", think about the positive results it will have on your brain. Let's see…Alzheimer's or NO Alzheimer's? I think I will memorize something!

If you are a sports enthusiast, you could memorize athlete's stats. If you like poetry, then poems. Politics, then your favorite political speeches. If movies, learn your favorite scenes, word for word. This tends to happen anyway, when we watch our favorite movies, over and over.

Some of my favorites are from the movie *Braveheart*. Some of the best lines for William Wallace (played by Mel Gibson, of course) is *"Every man dies. Not every man really lives."*

And *"They may take our lives, but they will never take our freedom."* Longshanks has a few good lines of his own like, *"The problem with Scotland is that it is full of Scots."*

I love the character of Princess Isabelle. She was a French princess forced to marry King Edward's (Longshanks) immature, evil, effeminate son for political alliance. In time, she falls in love with William. One of their first conversations is classic. I love it. Here it is:

Princess Isabelle: The king desires peace.

William Wallace: Longshanks desires peace?

Princess Isabelle: He declares it to me, I swear it. He proposes that you withdraw your attack. In return he grants you title, estates, and this chest of gold which I am to pay to you personally.

William Wallace: A lordship and titles. Gold. That I should become Judas?

Princess Isabella: Peace is made in such ways.

William Wallace: Slaves are made in such ways! The last time Longshanks spoke of peace I was a boy. And many Scottish nobles, who would not be slaves, were lured by him under a flag of truce to a barn, where he had them hanged. I was very young, but I remember Longshanks' notion of peace!

But, my favorite scene is when Longshanks is laying on his deathbed. William Wallace has been captured and is about to be tortured and executed for not swearing allegiance to King Edward (Longshanks). The French princess, Isabelle, enters the room, walks behind him, leans down low and whispers in his ear, while the beautiful music theme plays in the background,

"You see? Death comes to us all. But before it comes to you, know this: your blood dies with you. A child who is not of your line grows in my belly. You son will not sit long on the throne. I swear it!"

And she walks out. Of course, I'm standing up reciting every word with her in my best French accent.

Most of you can recite scenes, word for word, from your favorite movies. Besides **Braveheart**, I know all the lines for **Gone with the Wind** and **Sound of Music**. My husband knows all the words to **Terminator 2.**

The point is that everyone can **find something of interest to memorize**. No one is going to test you on it except yourself! Do it for your brain's health and have fun with it.

Of more importance, I love to memorize Bible scripture. It helps me in many ways. Memorizing scripture and meditating scripture go hand in hand. My personal belief is that it helps bring success in life, as it says in two of my favorite passages, which I memorized as a child.

"This Book of the Law shall not depart from your mouth, but you shall meditate in it day and night, that you may observe to do according to all that is written in it. For then you will make your way prosperous, and then you will have good success. Have I not commanded you? Be strong and of good courage; do not be afraid, nor be dismayed, for the LORD your God is with you wherever you go." Joshua 1:8-9

"But his delight is in the law of the LORD, and in His law he meditates day and night. He shall be like a tree planted by the rivers of water that brings forth its fruit in its season, whose leaf also shall not wither; and whatever he does shall prosper." Psalm 1:2-3

Each day I try to recall some of the scripture passages I've memorized. I continue to add new ones and spend time reviewing what I've learned before. This process helps me spiritually, mentally and even physically. I talk more about spiritual matters and Alzheimer's in a later chapter. **The point is to find something you love and memorize it. If it is something you are passionate about, you will relate emotion to it. Linking emotion, to a fact you are learning, builds even better and stronger neural networks.**

Chapter 7 Stress and Sleep

It's the bane of our society. Stress. Everyone has it to some degree. Often, it's overwhelming. Our bodies and brains show it. You don't need me to tell you how bad chronic stress is. You know it's bad for your body, but did you know it's also detrimental to your brain?

Deal successfully with stress and you may save your brain from dementia. If not, you could be setting yourself up for Alzheimer's disease. The following article from *sciencedaily.com* explains in more detail:

Repeated stress triggers the production and accumulation of insoluble tau protein aggregates inside the brain cells of mice, say researchers at the University of California, San Diego School of Medicine in a new study published in the March 26 *Online Early Edition of the Proceedings of the National Academy of Sciences.*

The aggregates are similar to neurofibrillary tangles or NFTs, modified protein structures that are one of the physiological hallmarks of Alzheimer's disease. Lead author Robert A. Rissman, PhD, assistant professor of neurosciences, said the findings may at least partly explain why clinical studies have found a strong link between people prone to stress and development of sporadic Alzheimer's disease (AD), which accounts for up to 95 percent of all AD cases in humans.

In the mouse models, we found that repeated episodes of emotional stress, which has been demonstrated to be comparable to what humans might experience in ordinary life, resulted in the phosphorylation and altered solubility of tau proteins in neurons," Rissman said. "These events are critical in the development of NFT pathology in Alzheimer's disease."

The effect was most notable in the hippocampus, said Rissman, a region of the brain linked to the formation, organization and storage of memories. **In AD patients, the hippocampus is typically the first region of the brain affected by tau pathology and the hardest-hit, with substantial cell death and shrinkage.**

Not all forms of stress are equally threatening. In earlier research, Rissman and colleagues reported that acute stress — a single, passing episode — does not result in lasting, debilitating long lasting changes in accumulation of phosphorylated tau. Acute stress-induced modifications in the cell are transient, he said, and on the whole, probably beneficial.

Acute stress may be useful for brain plasticity and helping to facilitate learning. **Chronic stress and continuous activation of stress pathways may lead to pathological changes in stress circuitry.** It may be too much of a good thing." As people age, perhaps their neuronal circuits do too, he said, becoming less robust and perhaps less capable of completely rebounding from the effects of stress.[1]

Another study showing stress to be a causative factor in Alzheimer's came from Finland. The *Dailymail.co.uk* web site gave this report.

Recent studies by Finnish researchers have found that the **long-term effects of stress may be the biggest cause of Alzheimer's disease.** When we are stressed, our blood pressure rises as a result of our heart beating faster, and the levels of cortisol in our blood stream also increase.

Dr. Nima Kivipelto and his colleagues from the University of Kuopio in Finland found that **patients with both high blood pressure and high cortisol levels were more than three times more likely to develop Alzheimer's disease than patients without these symptoms**.

In patients with **either** high blood pressure or high cortisol levels, **the risk was more than twice as likely.** Experts believe that once cortisol enters the brain, it starts to kill off brain cells, leading to Alzheimer's. **This suggests that stress is one of the largest causes of the condition**.

In fact, cases of Alzheimer's in the United States are now starting to appear in people in their forties and fifties — much younger than the expected age group to be affected by Alzheimer's. [2]

As you can see from these studies, it is absolutely essential that you establish healthy strategies to reduce chronic stress in your life. I consider myself an "expert" on this topic with good reason. Let me explain a small portion of my story.

In 2011, I had an unexpected life changing event. While walking my dogs in the springtime, I unknowingly picked up an infected deer tick. Within a few days I developed a severe case of Rocky Mountain Spotted Fever. I was put on 8 different antibiotics at one time while in the hospital. I was in and out of consciousness.

I was finally released from the hospital only to be re-admitted again within a week. After having yet another MRI, I was informed I had a previously undiagnosed pituitary tumor that would need to be treated once I was completely over the RMSF.

I was released again to go home and heal, but the healing did not come as expected. For three months, I threw up every day and was too weak to get out of bed. One more trip to a new endocrinologist brought another unexpected diagnosis.

After more blood work and reviewing all my medical records again (that about 100 doctors, literally, had already reviewed), this young endocrinologist said he knew what was wrong with me. His accurate conclusion was that the Rocky Mountain Spotted Fever had caused the pituitary tumor in my brain to hemorrhage and rupture. It literally "exploded" in my head. That would explain the bad headache. In the process, it "killed" the pituitary gland by cutting off all blood supply to it.

The pituitary gland is called the Master Gland. It controls almost all hormone function in your body, including one of the most important — cortisol, the major stress hormone. You cannot live very long without cortisol and I had already managed 3 ½ months, to the doctors amazement.

Stay with me here. This story directly relates to stress and the brain. After the office visit to the endocrinologist, I received a phone call from him late at night. He had just received the results of the blood work from earlier that day. I was shocked by what he said to me.

Try to imagine how you would react if your doctor said the following statement to you. "Melody, you cannot have ANY stress in your life! NO mental stress, NO emotional stress, NO physical stress, NO infections, NO injuries, period!"

My first response, while laughing in disbelief was, "But, I'm good as those things!" He said, "I'm not kidding. For you, stress can now become a life or death event. Because you no longer have a functioning pituitary (and therefore, no cortisol), your body literally cannot respond to stress. If you are injured, sick or stressed out and you do not get the right medicine in time, you can go into shock and could die within a few hours." He had my attention.

I wanted to tell him that what he just told me stressed me out a little bit! As I pondered this new situation and tried to imagine how I would manage it, I wondered how I would make this work. No stress at all??? What was I supposed to do — live in a bubble or a cave with no access to the modern world? Oh, I can't do that either, it would stress me out, too!

So, I cried a little bit and felt sorry for myself, and then realized I was not going to go into hiding or withdraw from the modern world. At first, I thought I could find a local support group on-line, but I found nothing. After digging up some statistics, I found that what happened to me only happens to *two people in a million!*

Gee! So much for a local support group! I was basically on my own. I had to find a way to make this new reality work and still be happy and healthy. By necessity, I would become a master of stress management.

I still had a long recovery ahead of me from the RMSF, and then I had to learn how to live with this new situation. The doctor said it was a permanent condition. Once the blood flow was cut off from the pituitary and it "died", there was no way for it to regenerate. The body will get rid of dead necrotic tissue. I dug around on-line for research regarding damaged pituitary. I could find no cases of a hemorrhaged pituitary regenerating and becoming functional again. I plan to be the first one.

In the meantime, if I was going to continue living, I absolutely had to learn effective ways to minimize daily stress in my life. I believe I've done a good job. In general, I am happier and healthier than most people I know. I still have to take my daily cortisone and other hormones. It has been a very interesting year with a few close calls. But, overall, I'm doing great!

So what do I do to manage stress? I'm going to talk about three of my favorite techniques here. There are many more that I use. I plan to write another book about effective stress management. Stay in touch with me by my web site www.nomorealzheimers.com or by following me on Facebook, to learn more and find out when my next book will be available.

Step one is to **recognize when you are feeling stress and deal with it right then**. When we experience frequent or chronic stress, we begin to think the tight neck and shoulders, headaches, stomachaches and a foul mood are normal. They are neither normal nor healthy. Before you will use a stress relieving technique, you have to recognize you are stressed and that it's time to take action.

Breathing is an automatic function and therefore, most people don't think about it. Autonomic breathing tends to be shallow, barely inflating the lungs. When we are under acute stress, the normal reaction is to gasp and hold our breath. One of the healthiest things you can do for your body is to pay attention to your breathing and learn to control it. Make it work for you.

Faced with chronic stress however, we may continue to do the same thing without knowing it. I realized I had been holding my breath for years and it took real effort to break that habit and learn to fully inhale and exhale again. **Controlling your breath is one of the easiest and most effective things you can do to relieve physical stress.** You will find that once you have calmed down, you will be able to think clearer. Here are some simple, but very effective exercises to get you started. Take control of your breath and you can take control of your health.

Deep Breathing

When you take time to breathe fully and slowly, you send signals to your brain that cause your entire body to relax. Additional benefits are lowered blood pressure, slowed heart rate, increased metabolism and sending life-giving oxygen to all of your organs, brain, muscles and cells. It's not hard. You just have to think about it in order to do it. I have *"Breathe"* signs in my house and on the steering wheel of my car. I also have one on my computer monitor since I spend much time there.

The goal is to breathe slowly and more fully, at least some time during the day. Make it a point to take some nice deep breaths. Then **SLOWLY** and fully exhale. The more you can do this during the day, the better, but especially when you are becoming stressed. Controlled deep breathing can also help you to fall asleep sooner and sleep better during the night. As you are slowly and fully inhaling and exhaling, relax your muscles, especially in the neck and shoulders. Think about relaxing your muscles from your face all the way down to your toes.

I'm getting sleepy just thinking about this. It works!

Other variations include holding your breath for a time period at the top of the breath (inhaling) and/or also, at the bottom (exhaling). For example, slowly inhale to the count of 4 (or 6 or 8). Hold that breathe for 4 counts. Slowly exhale to the count of 4 and hold for 4 counts.

You can also simply inhale slowly and deeply to count of 4 and then exhale slowly to count of 4. It's not hard. Some books and web sites try to make it complicated when it doesn't need to be. Just breathe!

Laughter and a Sense of Humor

Laughter is the best medicine. In college, *Anatomy of an Illness,* by Norman Cousins was required reading. A writer and medical researcher, Cousins found himself with a crippling disease. He used mega doses of Vitamin C, faith and laughter to help his body heal. He watched old movies of the Marx brothers. He reported, *"I made the joyous discovery that ten minutes of genuine belly laughter had an anesthetic effect and would give me at least two hours of pain-free sleep. When the pain-killing effect of the laughter wore off, we would switch on the motion picture projector again and not infrequently, it would lead to another pain-free interval."*

I try to find reasons to laugh every day. It helps to have four dogs and a cat. My husband calls them "cheap entertainment". Watching funny TV shows, such as *Everybody loves Raymond* and *America's Funniest Home Videos* is required in our home.

I limit the news and dramatic, violent TV shows. I've found I don't really miss anything. I still scan headlines on-line, and if I want to know more about something I can find it without having to watch all of the bad news. I like to get funny things by e-mail and Facebook. I pass them along and make someone else smile.

Medical research has come a long way since the time of Norman Cousins to document the benefits of laughter. Following is an article from the *Mayo Clinic* on this topic:

> Whether you're guiltily guffawing at an episode of "South Park" or quietly giggling at the latest New Yorker cartoon, laughing does you good. Laughter is a great form of stress relief, and that's no joke.
>
> A good sense of humor can't cure all ailments, but data is mounting about the positive things laughter can

do. A good laugh has great short—term effects. When you start to laugh, it doesn't just lighten your load mentally, it actually induces physical changes in your body. Laughter can:

—Stimulate many organs. Laughter enhances your intake of oxygen—rich air, stimulates your heart, lungs and muscles, and increases the endorphins that are released by your brain.

— Activate and relieve your stress response. A rollicking laugh fires up and then cools down your stress response and increases your heart rate and blood pressure. The result? A good, relaxed feeling.

— Soothe tension. Laughter can also stimulate circulation and aid muscle relaxation, both of which help reduce some of the physical symptoms of stress.

Laughter isn't just a quick pick-me-up, though. It's also good for you over the long haul. Laughter may:

— Improve your immune system. Negative thoughts manifest into chemical reactions that can impact your body by bringing more stress into your system and decreasing your immunity. In contrast, positive thoughts actually release neuropeptides that help fight stress and potentially more serious illnesses.

—Relieve pain. Laughter may ease pain by causing the body to produce its own natural painkillers. Laughter may also break the pain-spasm cycle common to some muscle disorders.

— Increase personal satisfaction. Laughter can also make it easier to cope with difficult situations. It also helps you connect with other people.[3]

Music

They say music soothes the savage beast. When we are under stress we may feel like the beast, and other times we feel like the beast is getting the best of us. Either way, music can help change our moods and relieve stress. If you are feeling down and tired, music can pick you up. If you are feeling riled up and anxious, music can help you relax.

We are a society plugged in. Most of us have music at our fingertips and ear buds in our head. In an earlier chapter I showed how playing a musical instrument can help build cognitive reserve. Research shows it can also relieve stress. Following is part of an interesting article from *Webmd.com:*

Stress starts in the brain and then kicks off a chain reaction that switches on the stress response in every cell of our bodies. Over time, these cellular switches can get stuck in the "on" position, leading to feelings of burnout, anger, or depression as well as a host of physical ailments.

Researchers now know that playing a musical instrument can switch off the stress response, improving physical and emotional health. When our senses detect a possible threat in the environment, the body undergoes a chain reaction in which genes within each cell switch on, directing the cells to produce chemicals associated with the stress response. Playing music sets off an opposite chain reaction that switches these genes off again.

Here's even better news: You don't have to be as proficient as violinist Joshua Bell to get the benefits; quite the opposite, in fact. The more seriously you approach musicianship, the less relaxing it may be.

Typical music-making is based on practice, performance, and mastery. In recreational music-making, our intention is to feel comfortable and nurtured in a creative experience with absolutely no pressure," says Barry Bittman, MD, CEO and medical director of Meadville Medical Center's Mind-Body Wellness Center, in Meadville, Pa.

What's the best way for the not-so-musically-inclined to get in the swing? Barry Bittman, MD, has some pointers:

Don't pick up a guitar. Mastering basic finger technique takes too long, Bittman says. Your goal is to enjoy the experience here and now. It's important to choose an instrument that doesn't require tons of technique to sound good. He suggests digital keyboards that let you make pleasant sounds just by pressing keys. Or just bang on a can.

Play by ear. Don't worry about learning songs or reading music. Instead, simply jam away for the fun of it.

Enjoy often. It does take time for the benefits of music-making to create lasting changes in your cells. **Studies have found that playing an hour a week for six weeks can lower the stress response**. Making music is like any other wellness activity; you should make it a permanent lifestyle change.[4]

Listening to beautiful, soothing, relaxing music can lower your blood pressure, heart rate and cortisol levels. That's a big plus for our health. Listening to soothing music before bed time can help you fall asleep faster and sleep longer. Find music you like and use it as a tool to benefit your health.

SLEEP

Like stress, sleep deprivation is common in our society. There is a connection between Alzheimer's and sleep. But, first let's look at the problem of sleep loss. *The Center for Disease Control (CDC)* has called it epidemic and a detriment to public health. Following is part of an article from the *CDC* concerning this important topic.

Sleep is increasingly recognized as important to public health, with sleep insufficiency linked to motor vehicle crashes, industrial disasters, and medical and other occupational errors. Unintentionally falling asleep, nodding off while driving, and having difficulty performing daily tasks because of sleepiness all may contribute to these hazardous outcomes.

Persons experiencing sleep insufficiency are also more likely to suffer from chronic diseases such as hypertension, diabetes, depression, and obesity, as

well as from cancer, increased mortality, and reduced quality of life and productivity. Sleep insufficiency may be caused by broad scale societal factors such as round-the-clock access to technology and work schedules, but sleep disorders such as insomnia or obstructive sleep apnea also play an important role. An estimated 50-70 million US adults have sleep or wakefulness disorder. Notably, snoring is a major indicator of obstructive sleep apnea. [5]

The body makes a multi-functional hormone called **melatonin,** known primarily for its ability to help us fall asleep. Like many other hormones, our melatonin levels decrease as we age. Many people have trouble falling and staying asleep because they lack melatonin. **There is also a connection between melatonin and Alzheimer's** as you will soon see. This portion of an article from the *National Sleep Foundation* explains how melatonin works:

The pattern of waking during the day when it is light and sleeping at night when it is dark is a natural part of human life. Only recently have scientists begun to understand the alternating cycle of sleep and waking, and how it is related to daylight and darkness.

A key factor in how human sleep is regulated is exposure to light or to darkness. Exposure to light stimulates a nerve pathway from the retina in the eye to an area in the brain called the hypothalamus. There, a special center called the supra-chiasmic nucleus (SCN) initiates signals to other parts of the brain that control hormones, body temperature and other functions that play a role in making us feel sleepy or wide awake.

The SCN works like a clock that sets off a regulated pattern of activities that affect the entire body. Once exposed to the first light each day, the clock in the SCN begins performing functions like raising body temperature and releasing stimulating hormones like cortisol. The SCN also delays the release of other hormones like melatonin, which is associated with sleep onset, until many hours later when darkness arrives.

Melatonin is a natural hormone made by your body's pineal gland. This is a pea-sized gland located just above the middle of the brain. During the day the pineal is inactive. When the sun goes down and darkness occurs, the pineal is "turned on" by the SCN and begins to actively produce melatonin, which is released into the blood. Usually, this occurs around 9 pm. As a result, melatonin levels in the blood rise sharply and you begin to feel less alert. Sleep becomes more inviting. Melatonin levels in the blood stay elevated for about 12 hours — all through the night — before the light of a new day when they fall back to low daytime levels by about 9 am. Daytime levels of melatonin are barely detectable.

Besides adjusting the timing of the clock, bright light has another effect. It directly inhibits the release of melatonin. That is why melatonin is sometimes called the "Dracula of hormones" — it only comes out in the dark. Even if the pineal gland is switched "on" by the clock, it will not produce melatonin unless the person is in a dimly lit environment. In addition to sunlight, artificial indoor lighting can be bright enough to prevent the release of melatonin.[6]

So what is the connection between sleep, melatonin and Alzheimer's? A report from *naturalnews.com* presents an additional link showing that **lack of melatonin and sleep may be a cause of Alzheimer's.** Following is a portion of that report:

Research suggests that a soluble form of amyloid beta, the main component of the plaques, may be a causative agent for Alzheimer's disease.

Several forms of treatment are indicated as possible interventions against the development of plaques, including strengthening the individual's immune system to trigger antibodies to prevent or clear plaques from the brain. **An important discovery was made indicating that the sleep hormone melatonin inhibits the formation of plaques and may be effective in the prevention of Alzheimer's; however, melatonin, cannot reverse the formation of existing plaques**, so is not useful in the treatment of the disease. Experiments in mice suggest that when adequate amounts of melatonin are available earlier in life, it may act to prevent Alzheimer's from developing.

Melatonin is a naturally produced hormone, which regulates sleep and the circadian rhythm of amyloid beta. People need enough melatonin to produce proper sleep, and excessive wakefulness reduces the amount of the hormone, leading the way to possible plaque development. Animal experiments also indicate the ability of melatonin to correct slight elevations in cholesterol, another risk factor for plaque development.

Excessive periods of sleep deprivation for any reason can affect the circadian rhythm of amyloid beta by reducing the amount of melatonin produced in the brain, hypothetically causing the buildup of amyloid beta plaque formation. **Recent findings have shown that chronic loss of sleep is connected to early onset Alzheimer's disease.**

It is possible to supply melatonin through supplementation; however, it is also possible to create additional quantities of melatonin without drugs or supplements. The pineal gland produces melatonin, whose quantities are stimulated by the presence of darkness and inhibited in the light. **Sleeping in a very dark room with no ambient light can stimulate melatonin production. Creating the conditions of twilight for several hours before going to bed will also set the stage for melatonin production and assist in falling asleep. Keep lights dim and remove all sources of light from the bedroom.**[7]

As this article points out, one way to naturally produce more melatonin is to lower lights several hours before bedtime. This simulates the sun going down and signals the brain to begin producing melatonin. You should become more relaxed and drowsy. Try to keep noise and light to a minimum.

Now that we know lack of sleep and melatonin can contribute to the development of Alzheimer's, what can we do to get a better night's sleep? I have several suggestions that most people do not do. Let's start with melatonin supplements.

Melatonin is a hormone. There is some controversy about its use as an over the counter product. It is available in various strengths. Most experts who recommend melatonin suggest 3-5 mg. about 30 minutes before bed. If you are older, you may do better with a larger dose of 10 mg. time released. I find this to be very helpful. It is also recommended to take a break from melatonin supplementation occasionally (maybe a few days to a week) and then resume it. This keeps the body from becoming de-sensitized to it.

As mentioned before, sleeping in a very dark room is mandatory for natural melatonin production.

Take a close look at your bedroom after you turn off the lights tonight. Give your eyes a few minutes to accommodate to the true light level. You will likely find light from some source in your room.

It may be coming from a nightlight in the hall shining under the door. Or, you may even have one in your room. Please turn it off and do not use night lights for yourself or your children. IT

WILL DISRUPT YOUR SLEEP AND SET A BAD PRECEDENT FOR YOUR CHILDREN!

When they get used to sleeping with a night light as a child, many continue to do so as adults. This is a very serious problem as a lack of melatonin has been associated not only with Alzheimer's, but also other diseases, including an increased risk of breast cancer.

Light can enter your room through a window from outside lights or the moon. You may need to install dark sleep shades. Lights from power buttons on computers, speakers, phones, etc. may be shining, as well. Most people have a lighted digital alarm clock. Ideally, you would not have a lighted alarm clock in your bedroom. If you do, at least turn it away from you at night. You don't need to lay awake in bed worrying about what time it is anyway! You could use an old fashioned clock with glow-in-the-dark hands that move (remember those?). Stores still sell them. Look for alternatives that won't interfere with your health.

Your eye lids are very thin. Light does penetrate them and registers on the retina. That's why the night lights and other light sources in the room still affect the production of melatonin even when your eyes are closed in sleep.

One of the best items I've found to promote good quality sleep is a **sleep mask**. I know this may seem like an old fashioned idea and few people use them now. However, it is an effective shield against light entering your brain through those thin eye lids.

I have tried many types over the years. I do not recommend cheap drug store masks. They are usually too small and don't fit well. Look for a sleep mask that is contoured and/or fully covers the entire eye area and fits well. You may have to try several to find the right one for you. It will be worth it. The one I use is called the "sleep master". It is available from amazon.com and other on-line retailers for about $25.00. It's a great investment for your health.

Your **pillow** can affect not only your sleep, but how you feel when you wake up. Most pillows simply do not provide sufficient support to the neck, head and shoulders. In the past, I used only contoured cervical pillows, also called orthopedic pillows. There are many types on the market, some cheap and some more expensive. My favorite orthopedic pillow is from a company called Foot Levelers. I like the pillow-pedic model. It sells for about $45.00 on Amazon.com. and is also found in many chiropractic offices.

The pillow manufacturers are finally getting the message that many of their pillows are not comfortable and do not provide needed support. Several companies are now making gusseted pillows that look and feel more like a traditional pillow, but actually provides support for the neck, head and shoulders, more like an orthopedic pillow. One of the best for the money I've found is from Beauty Rest. It is the Hotel luxury Firm model, available at Wal-mart for around $13.00. Not bad. For me it was very similar to the more highly priced "My Pillow" at about $70.00. "My Pillow" is a decent pillow also, and is available on-line at www.mypillow.com.

A good cervical pillow will support the head and neck. This allows the neck and shoulder muscles to relax and helps keep the cervical spine in alignment while you sleep. Your neck and shoulder muscles should feel good when you wake up. If not, then you may need a different pillow. Like the sleep masks, you may have to try a few to find one that fits you well. Again, this is totally worth the money and effort. It can make a huge difference in your sleep and well-being during the day.

Using a small pillow between your knees, if you sleep on your side, or a large pillow under your knees, if you sleep on your back, helps relax the hips and lower back. Your entire body will be more relaxed, promoting better sleep.

If these suggestions do not help you sleep better, please see your medical doctor for evaluation and possibly an overnight sleep study. This is important, especially if you snore. A good night's sleep is critical to your health and brain.

Chapter 8   Social and Spiritual Approaches to Brain Health

As we get older it is essential to stay socially connected to other people. Friends and family are important for reasons other than our emotional health. These social interactions are important for our brain health, and even in preventing Alzheimer's. One of the best research studies on this effect was done by *Rush University Medical Center*. Following is a portion of an excellent summary article explaining the research and results:

Having close friends and staying in contact with family members offers a protective effect against the damaging effects of Alzheimer's disease according to research by physicians at Rush University Medical Center in Chicago.

While other studies have shown people with more extensive social networks were at reduced risk of cognitive impairment, the study by Dr. David A. Bennett, and his colleagues from the Rush Alzheimer's Disease Center, is the first to examine the relations between social networks and Alzheimer's disease pathology.

Researchers studied elderly people without known dementia who are participating in the Rush Memory and Aging Project, an epidemiological and clinic-pathological study of aging and Alzheimer's disease that involves over 1,100 volunteers across northeastern Illinois. Brain autopsy was done at the time of death and post mortem data was available for analysis from the first 89 people.

Many elderly people who have the tangles and plaques associated with Alzheimer's disease don't clinically experience cognitive impairment or dementia," said Bennett. "Our findings suggest that social networks are related to something that offers a 'protective reserve' capacity that spares them the clinical manifestations of Alzheimer's disease."

Participants in the study underwent clinical evaluations and 21 cognitive performance tests each year. To determine social network, participants were asked about the number of children they have and see monthly. They were asked about the number of relatives, excluding spouse and children, and friends to whom they feel close and with whom they felt at ease and could talk to about private matters and could call upon for help. They were asked to specify how many of these people they see monthly. Their social network was the number of these individuals seen at least once per month.

The relationship between the amount of Alzheimer's disease pathology and cognitive performance changed with the size of the social network. As the size of the social network increased, the same amount of pathology had less effect on cognitive test scores. In other words, for persons without much pathology, social network size had little effect on cognition. **However, as the amount of pathology increased, the apparent protective effect on cognition also increased. Thus, social network size appears to have offered a protective reserve capacity despite the fact that their brains had the**

tangles and plaques indicative of Alzheimer's disease.[1]

Another summary article from *Alzheimer's Weekly* about this same study examined the risk of developing Alzheimer's if you stay lonely. This converse perspective noted an increase in risk for those who do not stay socially active. Following is a portion of this article:

> Being social may lower the risk of developing Alzheimer's disease later in life, new research suggests. Researchers at the Rush University Medical Center in Chicago assessed loneliness and dementia in 823 people, averaging almost 81 years of age, for up to four years. Seventy-six people developed Alzheimer's disease during the course of the study, which is published in the journal Archives of General Psychiatry.
>
> **According to the researchers, each point of increase on the loneliness score was associated with about a 51 percent increased risk of developing Alzheimer's.**[2]

Knowing that social interaction helps prevent Alzheimer's just makes sense to me. Based on other preventative measures, social interaction allows you to use more parts of your brain with stimulating conversation, recalling memories, as you discuss topics and laughing (stress relief) as you enjoy the company of others.

Spiritual

Dr. Caroline Leaf is a neuroscientist and author of the book, *Who Switched Off My Brain?* In this book, she discusses how our thoughts literally change the shape of our brains and how negative or "toxic" thoughts affect our mental, emotional and physical health. She states that according to medical research, up to 98% of all illnesses are a direct result of our thoughts.[3]

Toxic thoughts, coming from our reactions to stress and other events, create negative emotions, such as un-forgiveness, anger, bitterness, anxiety, worry and fear. These toxic thoughts and emotions cause a chemical cascade that ultimately weakens the body in numerous ways.

In her blog, Dr. Leaf described the results of a scientific study of emotions on DNA. She wrote the following:

> This study showed that thinking and feeling anger, fear and frustration caused DNA to change shape according to thoughts (that is thoughts with their intertwined feelings). **The DNA responded by tightening up, becoming shorter and switching off many DNA codes,** which reduced quality expression; we will feel "shut down" by negative emotions and our body feels this too.

What was really exciting about this study is the fact that the negative "shut down" or poor quality of the DNA codes was reversed with feelings of love, joy, appreciation and gratitude! The researchers also found that HIV positive patients with these positive thoughts and feelings had 300,000 times the resistance![4]

Dr. Leaf teaches how to take control of our thoughts and change dangerous toxic thinking. She explains that **our thoughts will literally change and restructure cells**. Toxic thoughts cause cellular changes that can allow disease to develop. However, **positive thoughts and emotions release chemicals that promote healing, memory formation and feelings of peace.**[5]

Un-forgiveness may be the most damaging toxic thought, according to Dr. Leaf. Harboring un-forgiveness against someone is like drinking poison and expecting the other person to die. It only hurts us. We greatly benefit, both in body and mind, by truly forgiving anyone who has wronged us. **We can literally protect our brain and heart by extending forgiveness.** Whatever we do to protect the brain slows deterioration and helps prevent Alzheimer's.

The purpose of this book is to demonstrate how properly nourishing and protecting the brain promotes optimal function and discourages the deterioration that leads to Alzheimer's.

The human brain is so complex and wonderful that we cannot fully comprehend it. The brain is the master director of all health functions. It allows us to think and feel emotions. It houses the imagination giving us the amazing ability to be creative.

In order to create, we have to see things in our **"mind's eye"**. Imagination can be used in positive ways, such as problem solving, creating beautiful art and music or designing new products. We also have the choice to use our imagination for unhealthy purposes such as undue fear, worry, anxiety, or even harming ourselves or someone else.

As a Christian, I believe God gave us imaginations to be used for good and healthy purposes. For example, imagination can help build your faith. Instead of "focusing" on my problems, I've learned to use the **"eyes of my heart"** and focus on my God and His provision for me. What does this have to do with preventing Alzheimer's?

I love to use my "holy imagination" or the "eyes of my heart" to see things in the Bible as being true in my life. For example, I love the 23rd Psalm. As I stated earlier in this book, it is one of the passages I quote each day to help keep my brain sharp and my faith strong.

I literally "see" each verse in my mind. I especially love the part where David, the writer says, "You anoint my head with oil". With my eyes of faith, I see the Lord pouring warm healing oil on the top of my head. I feel it soaking into my brain and taking the oil's healing power throughout my body. It's the most wonderful feeling and I know it produces real physical effects in my brain. (See previous chapter).

Many research studies have validated the power of the mind to produce healing effects through the usage of positive thoughts and mental pictures. Visualization is used by sports psychologists to help athletes improve performance. Why does it work? **Because seeing the picture in your mind literally stimulates your brain in the same way as the actual performance**.

Anyone can benefit from this phenomenon. I love combining my interest in physical health with spiritual growth. It provides a way of integration and wholeness as body, mind and spirit become congruent.

Over the years, I've developed many healing visualizations based on my Christian beliefs and the Bible. Obviously, not everyone will agree with what I do it. This is what I believe and what works for me.

I'm considering writing another book just on this topic. **I would show how to use the "eyes of your heart" to heal your body, mind and emotions**. It is very powerful. Using these Bible based mental videos, brings a deep sense of peace to body and mind. In the process your faith and hope are strengthened. Never underestimate the power of faith and hope! **If this is something that interests you, please drop me a note on my web site and let me know**.

I will end this chapter with another healing image for your brain and body. It's best to be in a comfortable relaxed position as you are reading this. If possible, take a minute to lower the lights, maybe light a candle.

You can do this with eyes closed or open. Whatever works best for you. This is one of my favorite healing visualizations. I use it to release healing for the pituitary in my brain. You can use it to promote healing in any part of your body.

I begin by picturing Jesus. I see him walking toward me. He has a huge smile on his face as he sees me. His eyes radiate warmth and love. He reaches for me and wraps his strong loving arms around me in the biggest best bear hug I've ever had. I feel the stress leave my body as I melt into His arms. He finally lets me go and we sit down together.

He asks what is troubling me. I tell him I need the pituitary gland in my brain to be healed and functioning as it should be. He raises his hands. I see the scars from the nails that held Him on the cross. Then, those scars begin to radiate a bright blue healing light. He reaches out His healing hands, radiating light, and places them on my head and holds them there. I feel an amazing warmth flowing from his hands into my brain. I focus on this feeling for several moments. Then he removes his hands from my head and hugs me again. "Don't ever forget how much I love you", he says. "I'm always with you. Keep believing, for it will be to you as your faith is. I love you!"

Any time I use this visual, I feel rested, peaceful, happy, hopeful and healthier. **That beats the socks off of being discouraged, depressed, sick and tired.** We don't change overnight. Keep working on it and moving forward. It takes time, persistence and patience. **But each time you do something positive for yourself, you are building momentum that will move you in the direction you want to go**.

Chapter 9 Putting It All Together

I hope by this point I've convinced you that **you can protect your brain and prevent Alzheimer's!**

Listed below is a summary of all the studies I cited showing a specific percentage of risk reduction. I was amazed to see it all put together. Technically, we can't add these percentages together because each study was different from the others. However, to see it all laid out gives me confidence that **I can protect my brain from degeneration and therefore, Alzheimer's.** Listed below, in order of appearance, are the action/behaviors studied, and the corresponding reduction of risk for developing Alzheimer's.

Maintain healthy weight throughout lifetime — **300%**

Drink fruit and vegetable juices 3 times per week— **76%**

Drink 2 cups of green tea per day — **50%**

Avoid excess carbs and insulin resistance — **65%**

Avoid high homocysteine levels by taking Vit. B-6, Vit. B-12 and folic acid — **50%**

Take Vitamin D daily— **77%**

Take an aspirin or Advil 4 times per week— **45%**

Exercise at least 2-3 times per week— **60%**

Control high blood pressure and cortisol from stress— **200%**

Have regular social interaction with friends and family— **51%**

Wow! And that is not including the other studies that showed either increased memory skills or a significant amount of risk reduction, but didn't give a percentage amount. Those activities included the following:

Eat berries, vegetables, nuts, spices and drink coffee daily for antioxidant value.

Eliminate trans fats and limit saturated fats.

Drink plenty of water daily.

Avoid diabetes type 2.

Add medium chain triglycerides in your diet (ex. Coconut oil).

Drink highly nutritious smoothies with fruits, vegetables, nuts, seeds and healthy oils.

Take Acetyl-L- carnitine and alpha lipoic acid daily.

Get good omega oils by eating fish and taking krill oil and DHA.

Challenge your brain daily by doing crossword puzzles, Sudoku, playing chess, playing brain games, memorization, reading to learn, play a musical instrument, learn a new language and new skills.

Learn to control stress.

Do deep breathing exercises.

Get good quality sleep for at least 7-8 hours per night.

Don't stay lonely.

Develop your spiritual life.

Live, love, laugh, forgive, be at peace with yourself, God and others.

It is not necessary to do all of these things. **We are not looking for perfection, just progress.** I am neither a purist nor a perfectionist. But, I have greatly altered my lifestyle to include many of these things daily. Some days I do better than others. That's OK. It takes time to make changes and develop a healthy lifestyle. **By sharing this information with your family and friends, I firmly believe that we can be the generation to stop Alzheimer's.**

Now we know what our parents, aunts, uncles and grandparents who suffered with Alzheimer's did not know. Let's make them proud.

Final Word

If you have enjoyed this book and learned something of value, or even just been inspired, please do three things for me. **First, go to Amazon.com. Pull up this book and write a short (or longer) book review for me. That will help more people to see this book. The more people who read it, the more who will know what to do to avoid this horrible disease.** Secondly, get on my web site and contact me and let me know what you thought about the book. **Thirdly, please pass this information along to your friends and family.**

Together, we can stop Alzheimer's.

Blessings,

Dr. Melody Jemison

www.nomorealzheimers.com.

www.alzheimerspreventionlifestyle.com

dr.melodyjemison@gmail.com.

References

Chapter 1 Introduction

1. WebMD. Drinking Juice May Stall Alzheimer's. Fruit and Vegetable Juice May Cut Alzheimer's Disease by up to 76%. Alzheimer's Disease Health Center. Accessed 8/1/2012. http://www.webmd.com/alzheimers/news/20060831/drinking-juice-may-stall-alzheimers.

2. Alz.org. Alzheimer's Association. 2012 Alzheimer's Disease Facts and Figures, The Journal of the Alzheimer's Association. March 2012; 8:131–168 Accessed 7/20/12. http://www.alz.org/alzheimers_disease_facts_and_figures.asp.

3. Omrf.org. Oklahoma Medical Research Foundation. Accessed 7/20/12. http://omrf.org/2007/04/10/new-study-zeroes-in-on-the-genetic-roots-of-alzheimers.

Chapter 2 What is Alzheimer's?

1. Nia.nih.gov. National Institute of Health's National Institute of Aging. Accessed 7/20/12. http://www.nia.nih.gov/alzheimers/topics/alzheimers-basics.

2. Wbur.org. Preparing For An Alzheimer's 'Tsunami'. Accessed 9/3/2012. http://www.wbur.org/2011/11/14/alzheimers-care-planning.

3. Agingsociety.org. Alzheimer's Disease and Dementia – a Growing challenge. www.againgsociety.org/agingsociety/pdf/alzheimers.

4. Time Magazine On-line. Exercise to Protect Aging Bodies and Brains. Accessed 8/1/2012. http://www.time.com/time/health/article/0,8599,1956619, 00.html.

Chapter 3   Nutrition

1. Sixwise.com. All the Health Risks of Processed Foods — In Just a Few Quick, Convenient Bites. Accessed 8/12/2012.
http://www.sixwise.com/newsletters/05/10/19/all-the-health-risks-of-processed-foods-in-just-a-few-quick-convenient-bites.htm.

2. Guardian.co.uk. Obesity in middle age increases risk of dementia, Diseases such as Alzheimer's almost four times as likely to affect people who are obese in middle age, new study shows. Accessed 9/24/2012. http://www.guardian.co.uk/science/2011/may/02/obese —more—likely—to—develop—alzheimers—disease.

3. Fi.edu.The Franklin Institute. Accessed 7/26/2012. http://www.fi.edu/learn/brain/micro.html.

4. US National Library of Medicine National Institutes of Health. Deborah Josefson. Foods rich in antioxidants may reduce risk of Alzheimer's disease. Accessed 9/24/2012.
http://www.ncbi.nlm.nih.gov/pmc/articles/PMC1176018/.

5. Alzheimer's Weekly. Pomegranate Juice Makes a Difference. Accessed 8/1/2012. http://alzheimersweekly.com/content/pomegranate-juice-makes-difference.

6. WebMD. Alzheimer's Disease Health Center. Accessed 8/1/2012. http://www.webmd.com/alzheimers/news/20060804/alzh eimers-apple.

7. WebMD. Drinking Juice May Stall Alzheimer's. Fruit and Vegetable Juice May Cut Alzheimer's Disease by up to 76%. Alzheimer's Disease Health Center. Accessed 8/1/2012. http://www.webmd.com/alzheimers/news/20060831/drin king-juice-may-stall-alzheimers.

8. Heart.org. Trans Fats. Accessed 9/24/12. http://www.heart.org/HEARTORG/GettingHealthy/FatsA ndOils/Fats101/Trans-fats_UCM_301120_Article.jsp.

9. CBN News. Health and Science. Brain Shrinkage? Trans Fats Link to Alzheimer's. Accessed 8/1/2012. http://www.cbn.com/cbnnews/healthscience/2012/March/ Brain-Shrinkage-Trans-Fats-Link-to-Alzheimers-/.

10. ABC Science. Saturated fats linked to Alzheimer's. Accessed 8/1/2012. http://www.abc.net.au/science/articles/2009/09/08/26795 89.htm.

11. Fisher's Center for Alzheimer's Research Foundation. Fish and nuts may ward off Alzheimer's. Accessed 8/1/2012. http://www.alzinfo.org/07/articles/prevention-and-wellness-103.

12. Journal of Alzheimer's Disease. Press Release- 4-June-2012 — High Blood Caffeine Levels in Older Adults Linked to Avoidance of Alzheimer's Disease. Accessed 8/2/2012. http://www.j-alz.com/press/2012/20120604.html.

13. Livestrong.com. Green Tea Extract and Alzheimer's. Accessed 8/2/2012. http://www.livestrong.com/article/364016-green-tea-extract-alzheimers/#ixzz22PKsXc00.

14. US National Library of Medicine National Institute of Health. Dehydration affects brain structure and function in healthy adolescents. http://www.ncbi.nlm.nih.gov/pubmed/20336685.

15. Mayoclinic.com. Diabetes and Alzheimer's Linked. Accessed 8/2/2012. http://www.mayoclinic.com/health/diabetes-and-alzheimers/AZ00050.

16. www.diabetesincontrol.com. New Type 3 Diabetes Discovered. Accessed 8/2/2012. http://www.diabetesincontrol.com/index.php?option=com_content&view=article&id=2582.

17. Mercola.com. Four Tablespoons of This "Brain Food" May Prevent Alzheimer's. Accessed 8/5/2012. http://articles.mercola.com/sites/articles/archive/2010/12/13/can-this-natural-food-cure-or-prevent-alzheimers.aspx.

Chapter 4 Supplements

1. Livestrong.com. Compare Multivitamins. Accessed 9/24/12. http://www.livestrong.com/article/297650-compare-multivitamins/.

2. Russell L. Blaylock, MD. Health and Nutrition Secrets. 2002. Page 323. Health Press. Albuquerque.

3. PubMed.gov. Memory loss in old rats is associated with brain mitochondrial decay and RNA/DNA oxidation: partial reversal by feeding acetyl-L-carnitine and/or R-alpha-lipoic acid. Accessed 8/4/2012. http://www.ncbi.nlm.nih.gov/pubmed/11854529.

4. PubMed.gov. Alpha-lipoic acid as a new treatment option for Alzheimer's disease — a 48 months follow-up analysis. Accessed 9/24/2012. http://www.ncbi.nlm.nih.gov/pubmed/17982894.

5. Livestrong.com. Alzheimer's and R-Alpha Lipoic Acid. Accessed 9/24/12. http://www.livestrong.com/article/548957-alzheimers-ralphalipoic-acid.

6. National Institute of Health Press Release. Folic Acid Possibly A Key Factor In Alzheimer's Disease Prevention. Accessed 8/6/2012. http://www.nih.gov/news/pr/mar2002/nia-01.htm.

7. Fisher Center for Alzheimer's Research Foundation. The latest in folic acid and Alzheimer's Disease. Accessed 8/6/2012. http://www.alzinfo.org/08/articles/prevention—and—wellness—89.

8. Newscientist.com. Low levels of vitamin B12 linked to Alzheimer's. Accessed 8/7/2012. http://www.newscientist.com/article/dn19184-low-levels-of-vitamin-b12-linked-to-alzheimers.html.

9. Ageworks.com. Protect Your Heart: Lower your Homocysteine. Accessed 8/7/2012. http://www.ageworks.com/information_on_aging/nutrition/vitaminb.shtml.

10. Cancer Treatment Centers of America. Study Suggests Vitamin D Screening and Appropriate Supplementation Indicated for All Cancer Patients. Accessed 8/8/2012. http://www.cancercenter.com/cancer-center-news/news/vitamin-d-supplementation.cfm.

11. PsychCental.com. Vitamin D Explored as Alzheimer's Treatment. Accessed 8/9/2012. http://psychcentral.com/news/2012/03/09/vitamin-d-explored-as-alzheimers-treatment/35774.html.

12. Ann Weiler C et al. Higher vitamin D dietary intake is associated with lower risk of Alzheimer's disease: a 7-year follow-up. Journal of Gerontology: Medical Science 2012; doi:10.1093/gerona/gls107.

13. Naturalnews.com.Vitamin D: How to Determine Your Optimal Dose. Accessed 9/26/2012. http://www.naturalnews.com/027345_Vitamin_D_exposure_sun.html

14. Heart-health-for-life.com. Krill Oil Benefits. Accessed 8/9/2012. http://www.hear-health-for-life.com/krill-oil-benefits.html.

15. Newsroom.ucla.edu.com. This is your brain on sugar: UCLA study shows high-fructose diet sabotages learning, memory — Eating more omega-3 fatty acids can offset damage, researchers say. Accessed 8/18/2012. http://newsroom.ucla.edu/portal/ucla/this-is-your-brain-on-sugar-ucla-233992.aspx.

16. Cnn.com. Dr. Sanjay Gupta: An aspirin a day to keep Alzheimer's away? Accessed 8/10/2012. http://articles.cnn.com/2002-09-24/health/otsc.alzheimers.aspirin_1_amyloid-plaque-anti-inflammatory-medications-alzheimer/2?_s=PM:HEALTH.

Chapter 5   Physical Exercise

1. Alzforum.org. Total Activity, Not Just Exercise, Keeps Mind Sharp. Accessed 8/13/2012. http://www.alzforum.org/new/detail.asp?id=3143.

2. Livestrong.com. Aerobic Exercise and the Brain. Accessed 8/13/2012. http://www.livestrong.com/article/386939-aerobic-exercise-the-brain/.

3. Mayoclinic.com. Preventing Alzheimer's – Exercise is still the best. Accessed 8/13/2012. http://www.mayoclinic.com/health/alzheimers/MY00002.

4. Livestrong.com. Does a lack of exercise affect Alzheimer's? Accessed 8/13/2012. http://www.livestrong.com/article/424389-does-a-lack-of-exercise-affect-alzheimers/.

5. Cellmedicine.com. Physical Exercise Stimulates Stem Cells to Create New Brain Cells. Accessed 8/14/2012. http://www.cellmedicine.com/physica-exercise-neurogenesis/.

Chapter 6   Cognitive Reserve and Brain Training

1. Alzinfo.org. Brain Scans Support Cognitive Reserve Theory for Preventing Alzheimer's. http://www.alzinfo.org/04/articles/prevention-and-wellness-24.

2. Psychcentral.com. Bilingual Skill May Protect From Dementia. http://psychcentral.com/news/2012/03/30/bilingual-skill-may-protect-fromdementia/36735.html.

3. Philly.com. Musicians' Brains Might Have an Edge on Aging. http://www.philly.com/philly/health/HealthDay667292_20 120802_Musicians__Brains_Might_Have_an_Edge_on_Aging.html.

Chapter 7   Stress and Sleep

1. Sciencedaily.com. Chronic Stress Spawns Protein Aggregates Linked to Alzheimer's. Accessed 8/22/2012. http://www.sciencedaily.com/releases/2012/03/1203261 60819.htm.

2. Dailymail.co.uk. How stress can trigger Alzheimer's, heart disease and infertility. Accessed 8/22/2012. http://www.dailymail.co.uk/health/article-136346/How-stress-trigger-Alzheimers-heart-disease-infertility.html.

3. Mayoclinic.com. Stress relief from laughter? Yes, no joke. Accessed 8/28/2012. http://www.mayoclinic.com/health/stress-relief/SR00034/NSECTIONGROUP=2.

4. Webmd.com. How Making Music Reduces Stress. Accessed 8/29/2012. http://www.webmd.com/balance/stress-management/features/how-making-music-reduces-stress.

5. Cdc.gov. Insufficient Sleep Is a Public Health Epidemic. Accessed 8/30/2012. http://www.cdc.gov/features/dssleep/.

6. National Sleep foundation. Sleep and Melatonin. Accessed 8/30/2012. http://www.sleepfoundation.org/article/sleep-topics/melatonin-and-sleep.

7. Naturalnews.com. Melatonin may prevent Alzheimer's disease — sleep your way to brain health. Accessed 8/30/2012. http://www.naturalnews.com/034742_melatonin_Alzheimers_brain_health.html.

Chapter 8   Social and Spiritual Aspects of Brain Health

1. Rush University Medical Center. Social Networks Protect Older Adults Against Damaging Effects of Alzheimer s Disease According to Rush Study. Accessed 9/3/2012. http://www.rush.edu/webapps/MEDREL/servlet/NewsRelease?id=751.

2. Alzheimersweekly.com. Social Activity Lowers Risk of Alzheimer's. Accessed 9/3/2012. http://alzheimersweekly.com/content/socia-activity-lowers-risk-alzheimers.

3. Drleaf.com. You are what you think: 75% — 98% of physical and mental illnesses come from our thought life. Accessed 9/5/2012. http://drleaf.com/blog/general/you-are-what-you-think-75-98-of-mental-and-physical-illnesses-come-from-our-thought-life.

4. Drleaf.com. You are what you think: 75% — 98% of physical and mental illnesses come from our thought life. Accessed 9/5/2012. http://drleaf.com/blog/general/you-are-what-you-think-75-98-of-mental-and-physical-illnesses-come-from-our-thought-life.

5. Dr. Caroline Leaf. Who Switched Off My Brain? Revised edition e-book . Chapter 2. Thomas Nelson Publishers, 2009.

Made in the USA
Lexington, KY
29 April 2013